SURGICAL PATHOLOGY TECHNIQUES

D.G. Lowe
MD MIBiol MRCPath
Senior Lecturer/Honorary Consultant
Department of Histopathology
St Bartholomew's Hospital, London

I.J.M. Jeffrey
BSc MB ChB
Senior Registrar
Department of Histopathology
St Bartholomew's Hospital, London

B.C. Decker Inc.
Philadelphia • Toronto

Publisher

B.C. Decker Inc.
3228 South Service Road, Burlington, Ontario L7N 3H8

B.C. Decker Inc.
320 Walnut Street, Suite 400, Philadelphia, Pennsylvania 19106

Sales and Distribution

United States and Puerto Rico
Mosby-Year Book Inc.
11830 Westline Industrial Drive, Saint Louis, Missouri 63146

Canada
Mosby-Year Book Ltd.
5240 Finch Ave. E, Unit 1, Scarborough, Ontario M1S 5A2

Surgical Pathology Techniques **ISBN 1-55664-297-0**

Published in the United Kingdom by Wolfe Medical Publications Ltd 1990
Printed by Hazell Books Ltd, Aylesbury, England

Library of Congress catalog card number: 90-080929
10 9 8 7 6 5 4 3 2 1

Contents

Preface 4

Introduction 5

1 **Alimentary tract** 10
- Small specimens: Biopsies, polyps, small lengths of bowel wall 10
- Oesophagus 15
- Stomach 18
- Appendix and Meckel's diverticulum 21
- Small and large bowel 25

2 **Liver, gall bladder and pancreas** 31
- Liver 31
- Gall bladder 33
- Exocrine pancreas 36

3 **Female genital system** 40
- Vulva 40
- Cervix 44
- Uterine corpus 48
- Fallopian tube 55
- Ovary 57
- Fetus and placenta 60

4 **Breast** 64
- Biopsies 64
- Large specimens 65

5 **Male genital system** 74
- Testis 74
- Epididymis and vas 75
- Prostate 77
- Penis and scrotum 80

6 **Urinary tract** 82
- Kidney 82
- Ureter 87
- Bladder 87

7 **Respiratory system** 92

8 **Skin** 97

9 **Lymphoreticular system** 101
- Lymph nodes 101
- Spleen 102
- Bone marrow 105
- Thymus 105

10 **Endocrine system** 106
- Pituitary gland 106
- Adrenal gland 106
- Thyroid gland 110
- Parathyroid glands 115
- Endocrine pancreas 117

11 **Head and neck** 119
- Ear, nose, oral cavity and larynx 119
- Salivary glands 122

12 **Osteoarticular system and soft tissues** 124
- Bone and cartilage 124
- Lesions of joints and para-articular tissues 127
- Soft tissues 132

13 **Cardiovascular system** 133
- Small specimens 133
- Large specimens 134

14 **Central nervous system and eye** 136
- Brain and meninges 136
- Peripheral nerves 136
- Eye 137

Index 141

PREFACE

Diagnostic histopathology is largely an apprenticeship, learned through experience and by demonstration and example. The laboratory process begins with the macroscopical description and dissection of specimens received from theatre (the 'cut-up'), and it is at this stage that blocks of tissue for macroscopical examination are selected and taken. These techniques are usually learnt at an early stage in the histopathologist's career, by observing experienced members of staff and by practising under supervision.

This illustrated book is intended to help this learning process and is aimed primarily at the trainee histopathologist. It should continue to be of use to the pathologist once the basic techniques have been mastered, as even after practising for some time he or she is likely to receive specimens that have not been encountered before. Surgeons, gynaecologists and other clinicians would also greatly benefit from some knowledge of what happens to a specimen once it has left their hands.

These pages provide guidance on how to approach the preparation and dissection of a surgical specimen to demonstrate the pathology present. It also gives advice on the structuring and contents of macroscopical reports, and examples of these are paired with colour illustrations of the relevant specimens. Much of the descriptive and procedural data has been tabulated and highlighted to make the book easier to use at the dissection bench. Although the number and types of blocks taken in different laboratories may vary, in general the same principles of sampling can be applied; line drawings of the photographs are provided to indicate where blocks of tissue should be taken for microscopical examination.

We would like to acknowledge the help of Mr J.L. Hopwood, Museum Conservator at the Pathology Museum, St Bartholomew's Hospital, London, who took almost all of the colour photographs in this book. Figures 34-36 are reproduced by kind permission of Professor J. Jass of the University of Auckland (formerly of St Mark's Hospital, London). Figure 78 is reproduced by kind permission of Professor C.L. Berry of the London Hospital, the editor of the *British Medical Journal*, and the editor of the *Journal of Clinical Pathology*.

INTRODUCTION

The work of the surgical pathologist starts in the cut-up room, where specimens are identified, logged in, examined, described, dissected and prepared for histological processing. The purpose of the gross examination is to establish what the specimen consists of, what it looks like (and feels like, in many cases), and how it differs from normal. The components of the macroscopical report are therefore the specimen type (e.g. mucosal biopsy, hysterectomy, laryngectomy) or the tissues present (e.g. pericardium, small bowel diverticulum); measurements of the specimen (e.g. size, number and weight); a description of the pathology and of other tissues present; and, from large specimens, a description of the blocks of tissue taken for histological examination, with a record of the sites from which they were obtained and their numbers.

Specimen identification

Specimen identification is clearly a crucial part of the initial examination of a pathological specimen. The first sign of a mix-up of specimens will emerge at this stage. The clinical details on the request form should indicate the types and numbers of specimens, and these should be appropriate for the specimen received.

The pathological report identifies the surgical procedure that was performed or the tissues that were removed, and may be the only record of the operation if the case notes are lost. As the size and weight of the organ or tissue removed are recorded, it also provides a record of the extensiveness of the surgical procedure.

Photography has proved to be an excellent way of identifying a resection specimen and recording its macroscopical features. Colour photography should be used if possible, but good results can be obtained with monochrome Polaroid instant prints or black-and-white reel film. In complicated dissections (such as a laryngectomy or a Whipple's operation specimen), a second print can be used to mark the positions of the blocks of tissue taken and can greatly facilitate the macroscopical and microscopical reporting. Photography of fresh tissue has the particular advantage that the colours are preserved but there are several practical constraints, particularly the hazards to staff from infection and the need for staff and equipment to be available throughout the day, which may well limit feasibility. No such limitations affect the use of fixed specimens, so these are more likely to be used for photographic records, especially in a busy department.

Fixation

Most specimens are received fixed in 10 per cent formalin solution, though some tissues may be sent to the histopathology department fresh. Fresh material is needed for the following purposes:

- frozen section
- immunocytochemistry
- hormone receptor estimation and other biochemical studies
- cytological examination
- microbiological sampling before histopathology
- chromosome analysis
- research
- museum display.

Occasionally, specimens will be sent unfixed because they will not fit into a pot (e.g. a lower limb) or, in complicated cases, because a fresh specimen is necessary for satisfactory orientation and dissection.

When the above points have been dealt with, the tissue should be fixed before dissection. If suitable, the entire specimen should be fixed in as intact a state as possible, so that the relations between its parts are preserved. Some specimens, such as hollow organs, cysts, and masses of adipose tissue, will not fix well because the diffusion of fixative into the centre of the specimen will be delayed, but where cuts must be made to aid fixation, distortion of the specimen should be kept to a minimum. These cases will be discussed in the appropriate chapters.

Macroscopical description

The macroscopical report of a specimen records the gross features of the tissue received in the pathology department, and serves several important functions. With all specimens, but especially with biopsies, the report provides a check that the histological slides which are eventually prepared are representative of the tissue supplied, in both the number and the area of fragments. With a large resection specimen, the macroscopical description is usually the only recorded evidence of its appearance before it was cut, separated, dissolved or otherwise distorted for examination purposes. A good description of a specimen is therefore essential.

Some diagnoses are made principally from the macroscopical features; for example, cholelithiasis and sialolithiasis can be macroscopical diagnoses. The gross appearance of the specimen may also influence the final diagnosis, as with the distribution of lesions in the differential diagnosis of Crohn's disease and ulcerative colitis. If by mishap the blocks are embedded incorrectly or if the sections prove difficult to interpret, the macroscopical report may be the only means of diagnosing whether a tumour extends to an excision line or involves a serosal surface.

The report recording the appearance and other physical characteristics of a pathological specimen may also be of interest to clinicians, especially when the lesion has been seen, for example, at laparotomy or through an endoscope or laparoscope. Gynaecologists will probably be more interested to learn that a fibroid weighed 5 kg than to have it confirmed that it was indeed histologically diagnosable as a leiomyoma. The site of occurrence of a particular disease can be important for epidemiological studies and is usually defined, at least in part, in the macroscopical description. For forensic purposes, a record that an organ or part of one has been excised can occasionally be of value, for example, in helping to identify a cadaver.

Macroscopical descriptions should be short but they must contain all the salient details of a case. The active voice 'The kidney shows . . .' is generally preferable to the passive '. . . is found in the kidney', and in most cases the present tense is most suitable.

Estimation of the size of a lesion by comparison with familiar objects should be avoided. Oranges, eggs and peas, for example, come in a range of sizes, and if a report has to be sent overseas the original inexactitude may well be exaggerated. Measurements are usually given in centimetres (i.e. 3.7 cm rather than 37 mm) unless the specimen is very small, in which case millimetres can be used.

Weight is often an important descriptive parameter, especially when dealing with endocrine organs. When the average weight of the normal organ is known (or can be found in reference books), the weight of the abnormal organ may be significant, and may give some indication of the size or extent of the abnormality. Even when the normal weight is very variable, as for the prostate, the specimen weight can indicate whether a resection was modest or extensive. The significance of the weights of some tissues, such as mastectomy specimens or hysterectomy specimens, is more doubtful, though they may give a general indication of size.

When a tissue such as the endometrium or prostate is biopsied randomly or diffusely, the number of pieces tends to be unimportant, and the volume of the aggregated pieces gives a better impression of sampling. Directed biopsies such as endoscopic or colposcopic biopsies should be counted, to confirm the number of specimens received and to indicate the number of fragments that should appear on the histological sections. When biopsies are taken from different sites in an organ they must be labelled separately.

After fixation in formalin most tissues lose their natural colours and become grey or brown. Nevertheless, some idea of the colour is useful, especially when different parts of a tumour are differently coloured, since this may indicate that more than one tissue, host response, growth pattern, etc., is present. The same is true of differences in the consistency of the tissue and the texture of the surface.

Descriptive terms should not be too obscure. Clinicians are unlikely to reach for their dictionaries when faced with *grumous* or *pultaceous*, and the meaning of the report

Table

	DESCRIPTIVE TERMS	INTERPRETIVE TERMS
Colour	Red, clear, grey	Haemorrhagic, mucoid, necrotic
Contour	Round, irregular, ill-defined	Encapsulated, invasive, infiltrative
Consistency	Hard, soft, rubbery, gelatinous	Bony, calcified, necrotic, mucoid, fibrosed
Texture	Granular, fibrillary, smooth	Ulcerated, fibrinous
Size	Usually in centimetres; in millimetres for tiny objects	Enlarged, atrophic

may be obscured by such words. Pathologists' terms can be divided broadly into two groups: those which qualify the physical appearance of the specimen alone (descriptive terms); and those which draw from the physical appearances some conclusion about their nature (interpretive terms) (**Table**).

Morphological features can usually be described with impunity, since they can be appreciated by most people. For example, a tumour may be described as pink, well circumscribed, and hard, and unless the prosector is colour-blind or careless, the description is unlikely to be mistaken. Interpretive terms, on the other hand, may cause problems. The same tumour could be described by one prosector as an encapsulated, bony mass with areas of fibrosis, and by another as calcified tumour tissue which compresses the adjacent tissues. Interpretive terms may be admissible, however, when there is no doubt that haemorrhage, necrosis etc. has occurred.

Some terms have been used in specific contexts for many years and cannot now be used generally because of their associations. For example, if a soft grey or yellow area of tissue is described as *caseous*, clinicians may assume that tuberculosis is present; *waxy* is very rarely used, except to describe amyloidosis.

It is helpful to both pathologist and clinician if a report follows a logical sequence or progression. For the former, this provides a framework or check-list so that dissection progresses more quickly. The latter will be able to find points of interest more easily. Examples of sequences in common use (the direction of the sequence is not important) are as follows:

Vagina/cervix/endometrium/myometrium/fallopian tubes/ovaries;
Oesophagus/fundus/body/antrum/pylorus/duodenum.

For other specimens, the different aspects may provide a framework:

Mucosa/cut surface of wall/serosa/attached tissues;
External surface/cut surface/contents.

If the specimen has an obvious lesion such as a carcinoma, however, it would be irritating if its description was to be submerged by an academic sequence. In such a case, the carcinoma and the tissue where it arises should be described first, and the sequence used in a subsequent paragraph to remark on the other tissues present.

Principles of dissection

Dissection will depend on the tissues present in the specimen and on the type of organ or tissue received; whether it is intact or opened in theatre; whether it is fresh or fixed; the nature of the pathology; and whether this can be identified with certainty at an early stage in the procedure. The general principles of dissection are that all of the pathology should be assessed, that the features of prognostic importance should be noted, and that there should be as little distortion and destruction of the specimen as possible. This last principle is important if it becomes necessary to demonstrate the case to a clinician or to another pathologist, or to return to a particular area of the specimen in order to take more blocks.

On the whole, the procedures used to dissect the specimen are not detailed on the macroscopical report. It is not usually of interest to clinicians that, for example, 'The mesentery was then incised at 1 cm intervals . . .' or 'The stomach was opened along the greater curve . . .'. On the other hand, one might record that 'Despite a prolonged search for lymph nodes in this specimen, only two were found'.

Blocks

In the scope of this book it is possible only to give a general suggestion of the number of blocks which might be taken in any particular case. Obviously the exact number will depend on many differing factors, such as the size and complexity of the specimen, the research interests of the histopathology department, the forensic or legal implications of the case, and the individual practice and experience of the pathologist who is responsible for the surgical reporting. In the USA, for example, it is customary to take more blocks from certain specimens than is usual in the UK. If there is any doubt the advice of a senior staff member must be sought.

The size of the blocks of tissue taken from large specimens will be limited by the size of the processing cassettes in which they will be placed. In general, they should not be more than 4 mm thick and should not fit tightly into the cassette, so that diffusion of processing fluids into the tissues is not impeded.

The gross assessment of a case will determine which blocks are taken for preservation in the department's files. When a case is reviewed some time after initial reporting, the macroscopical description may be the only indication of the sites from which the blocks were taken. For example, if a resection specimen was found to have a focal lesion, the original description could serve to explain why no blocks were taken from some areas, and why numerous blocks were taken from a particular area.

In many cases, microscopical diagnoses cannot be made if the tissue submitted for processing is wrongly selected. For example, tissue from the periphery of a large bowel neoplastic polyp which does not include submucosa may prevent the histologist confirming or refuting a diagnosis of carcinoma.

In recording the sites of blocks, some degree of orientation will usually be necessary. The site of origin of the tissue may be important, and the way that it is embedded and sectioned may need to be specified. The parts of the block, such as resection margins, should be clearly identifiable.

Depending on the pathology present, standard blocks in addition to the lesion itself might include lymph nodes, samples of the tissue away from the lesion, vascular pedicles and resection margins.

The site from which a block is taken is usually recorded by giving the block an identifying letter or number (the back of the request form could be used for the record):

A	cord of tissue attached to mucosa
B	small polyp
C	large polyp
D	carcinoma
E	lymph nodes adjacent to tumour
F	distant lymph nodes
G	lymph nodes at highest point
H	proximal excision end
J	distal excision end.

The orientation of the tissue in the wax block is of great importance. It will determine which aspect of the tissue is lost when the block is trimmed ready for sectioning, which aspect of a lesion is cut and mounted on a slide, and the relationship of tissue components such as epidermis and dermis on the sections. Incorrect embedding may make a case unreportable, though fortunately the orientation of most blocks will be obvious to the experienced staff responsible for the embedding. If the orientation of a tissue in the block is critical, suitable directions should be recorded. Phrases in common use include:

- **On end** for a cord of tissue such as an artery or vas deferens (block A, above);
- **On side** when a cord or strip of tissue is not to be embedded on end;
- **On edge** when a flat sheet of tissue is from a hollow viscus and the layers of the wall are to be displayed (blocks H and J, above);
- **Cut side down** when an irregular, spherical or cylindrical specimen is bisected (blocks B, C, E, F and G, above).

Flat blocks (e.g. block D, above) are placed

into cassettes so that the face which is to be trimmed and sectioned first is downwards, away from the lid. In blocks H and J above further orientation might be necessary to identify which aspect of the block represents tissue at the excision lines.

Marking of the specimen with insoluble pigment may be essential in some cases, especially when the tissue may be distorted or fragmented by processing. There are several possible markers, the most commonly used being carbon particles from India ink, which can be carefully painted onto the surfaces to be identified and blotted dry. There is a risk that when a tissue is cut carbon will be carried into it on the knife blade but in practice this is seldom a problem. Other pigments which have been successfully used include alizarin crimson and viridian. When fresh specimens are received, inking of the excision margins and other important structures should where possible be done before fixation so that any distortion from fixation or processing can be allowed for. Blocks may also be marked with a notch or incision on the border away from or opposite the excision margin.

Decalcification

Tissues may be very hard or have focal gritty areas. If foreign material can be excluded, this means that the tissue is almost certainly calcified and will need decalcifying before routine processing. Common specimens which contain foci of calcification or fragments of bone include:

- nasal polyps
- apical granulomas and other dental specimens
- bone marrow aspirates
- some ovarian tumours
- meningiomas
- craniopharyngiomas
- areas of fat necrosis
- breast lesions
- products of conception
- intervertebral discs.

The staff responsible for the embedding should be warned if there is the possibility that calcium or bone may be present because of the damage that these cause to microtome blades, and to the surrounding tissues when the sections are cut. Before a specimen is decalcified, any special stains that might be needed should be discussed with the staff; some, such as methyl green pyronin stain for RNA, will not work well on sections which have already been decalcified with formic acid. Decalcification with EDTA chelates iron salts and makes Perls' stain unreliable.

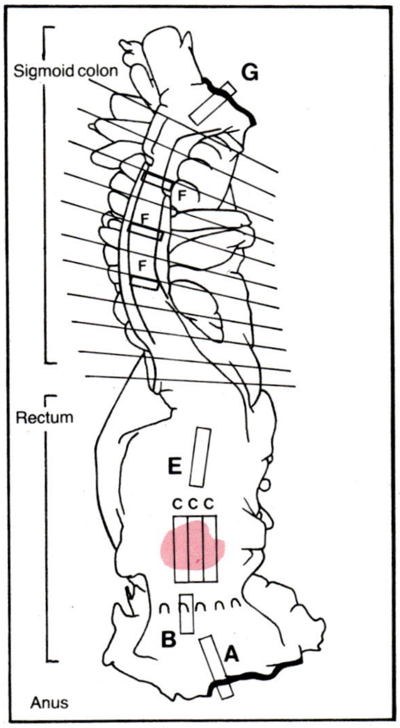

Key to illustrations

In the ensuing chapters line drawings of specimens, paired with photographs, are used to illustrate where blocks should be taken for microscopic examination. Figure 28b shown here is representative of the diagrammatic style.

Pathological lesion

Resection margin

Cuts into specimen at dissection

Blocks of tissue taken from specimen

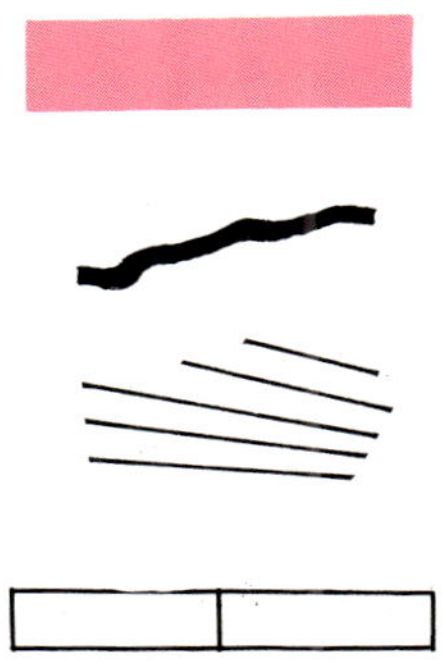

CHAPTER 1
ALIMENTARY TRACT

Small specimens

Biopsies

Biopsies from the alimentary tract are among the commonest specimens received by general histopathology laboratories. In most cases, fragments of tissue from different parts of the tract are handled in the same way. When several biopsies are received from one patient, the site of each must be specified in the report. This is made easier if the clinician uses a schematic drawing of the oesophagus, stomach or bowel and marks the biopsy sites on it (**1**).

Endoscopic mucosal biopsies are taken from almost anywhere in the tract but especially from the oesophagus, stomach, duodenum, terminal ileum and large bowel to investigate ulcers, neoplasms, diffuse and focal inflammation, and malabsorption. The biopsies are usually small and difficult to orientate. Jejunal biopsies taken by Crosby capsule for the investigation of small bowel disease are somewhat larger, but can become contracted and distorted. Where possible, biopsies are embedded at right angles to the luminal surface so that the sections will show the full thickness of the mucosa and include any submucosa that is present in the biopsy (**2**).

In some hospitals the gastroenterologists and surgeons arrange the biopsies mucosa upwards on small sheets of card before fixation. Strips of ruled cellulose acetate are very useful (**3**), since the biopsies can be placed along a line and the tissue and acetate processed, embedded and sectioned together. Distortion of the tissue is minimized and the sites of the biopsies can easily be identified by their position along the strip.

Small mucosal biopsies rarely need dissection or a detailed macroscopical description. Biopsies from the small bowel should be examined under a dissecting microscope before processing, to assess the villous pattern and check the orientation of the specimen if it is received attached to card or acetate sheet (**4**). Mishaps can sometimes occur; the specimen may be placed with the mucosal side downwards on the card, and the flat surface of the upward-facing muscularis mucosae or submucosa may be mistaken under the dissecting microscope for total villous atrophy.

The clinical details supplied with a case may indicate that levels or special stains will be needed. These should be asked for at the time of macroscopical reporting to avoid delay. If there is any doubt about the orientation of a specimen, however, it is best to begin by examining a single section. Otherwise the entire specimen may be lost by cutting multiple sections in the wrong plane.

Biopsies: Macroscopical report

Site	Oesophagus, stomach, duodenum, etc.
Type of specimen	Mucosal biopsy, tissue fragment, friable material
Measurements	Number of fragments Size, range of sizes or greatest dimension if very small
Description	Colour Whether attached to card or acetate

Polyps: Macroscopical report

Site	Rectum, sigmoid colon, etc.
Type of specimen	Sessile or pedunculated polyp(s)
Surgical additions	Suture markers, clips
Measurements	Diameter of head (pedunculated) or dimension of whole polyp (sessile) Length and diameter of pedicle if present Width of cuff of uninvolved tissue if present
Description	Colour Contour (villous, lobulated, smooth) Cut surface (cystic, papillary, solid)

Polyps

Polyps are circumscribed masses extending above the adjacent surface and may be pedunculated or sessile (**5**, **6**). They may be the result of a variety of pathological processes, such as inflammation, traction, hyperplasia, metaplasia or neoplasia. Histological examination is needed to establish the type of polyp and in neoplastic polyps to assess the extent of spread of neoplasia and the adequacy of the surgical excision.

Small polyps can be embedded whole, and if necessary multiple levels can be cut to display the stalk. Larger sessile polyps and pedunculated polyps with wide stalks can be bisected and embedded to show the cut surface (**5b**). If a polyp has a slender pedicle it should not be bisected since the very thin strand of tissue would tend to curl and distort. In this case, the head should be cut into three or more longitudinal blocks with a central block bearing the uncut pedicle (**6b**).

Small lengths of wall

Narrow rings or 'doughnuts' of wall can be taken from the excision margins and sent separately from a resection specimen (**7a**). Full thickness biopsies of bowel wall may also be taken for the investigation of Hirschsprung's disease. The dissection of an excised Meckel's diverticulum is described below (p 21).

The specimens should be measured and any abnormality of the mucosa, cut surface of wall or serosal surface recorded. If the doughnut is more than about 0.5 cm long, longitudinal blocks can be taken (**7b**). Thinner specimens should be divided into three or four pieces and embedded transversely.

Small lengths of wall: Macroscopical report

Site	Oesophagus, stomach, ileum, colon, etc.
Type of specimen	Ring (doughnut), sheet/strip of bowel wall
Measurements	Length and circumference, or area and thickness if a sheet of bowel is received
Surgical additions	Suture markers, clips, staples
Description	
Focal lesions	Ulcer, polyp, diverticulum
Rest of specimen	Mucosa, cut surface of wall and serosa: colour (red, purple, pale, etc.); consistency (friable, firm, fibrosed); contour (ulcerated, distorted, polypoid, fibrinous)

1

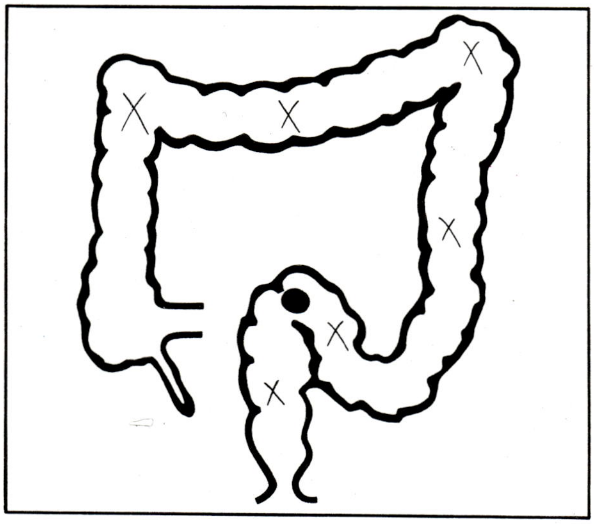

1 Diagram of the large bowel (made by a rubber stamp) on which the gastroenterologists have marked the sites from which a metaplastic polyp (●) and six biopsies (**X**) were taken. This method allows easy correlation of the pathological findings with the clinical features.

2

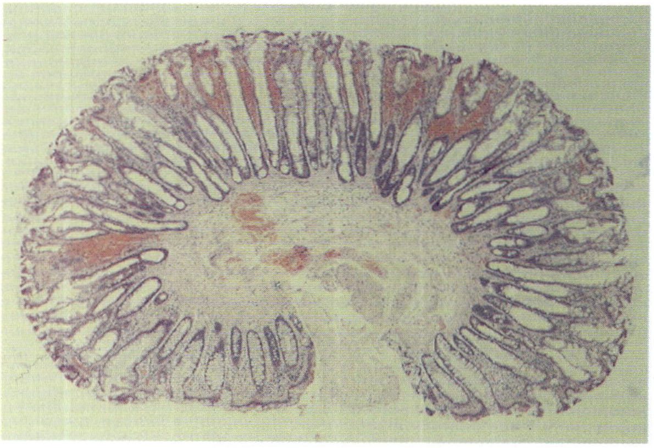

2 Histological section of a well-orientated rectal biopsy showing a metaplastic polyp. The relation between the mucosa and submucosa is clearly demonstrated.

3

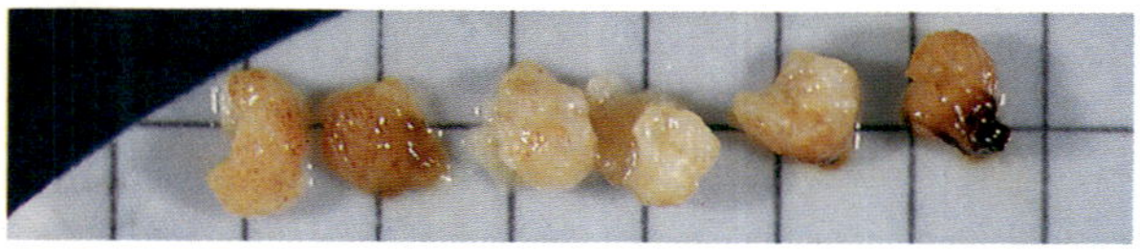

3 Large bowel biopsies arranged on a cellulose acetate strip in the same sequence as in **1**. The pointed end of the strip, by convention, indicates the most proximal biopsy, in this case from the hepatic flexure.

4

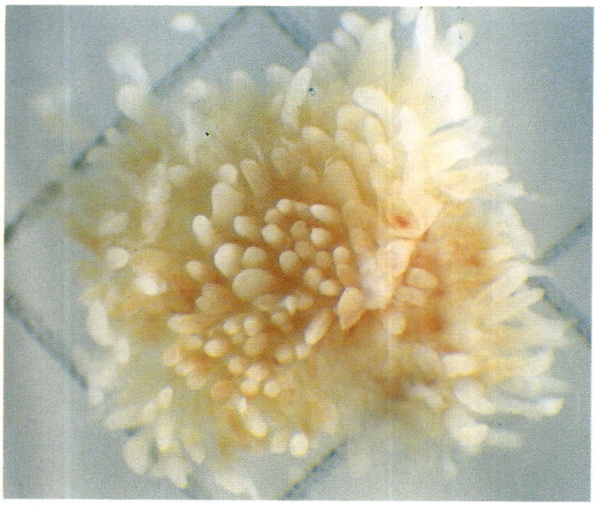

4 Small bowel mucosa viewed under a dissecting microscope in order to investigate malabsorption. The microscope reveals normal finger-like villi.

5a

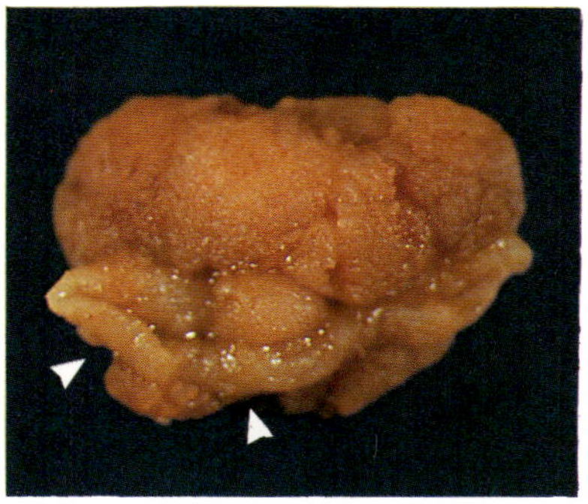

5b

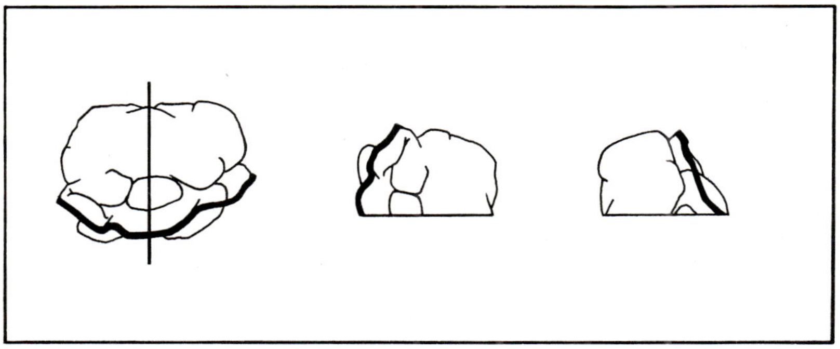

5a A sessile polyp of the large bowel surrounded by a short skirt of normal large bowel mucosa (▶).

5b A sessile polyp bisected and both halves embedded cut side down.

6a

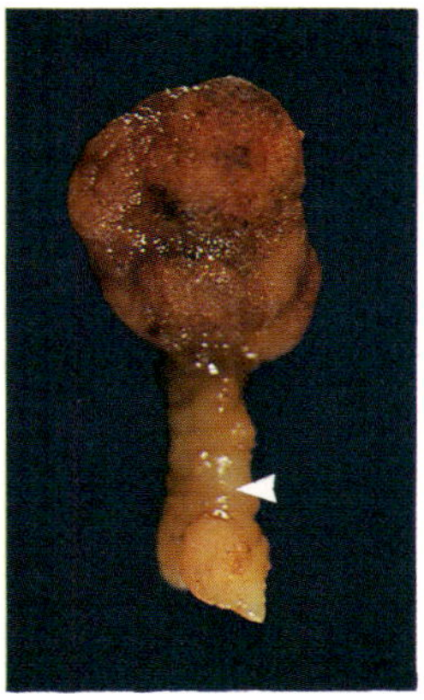

6b

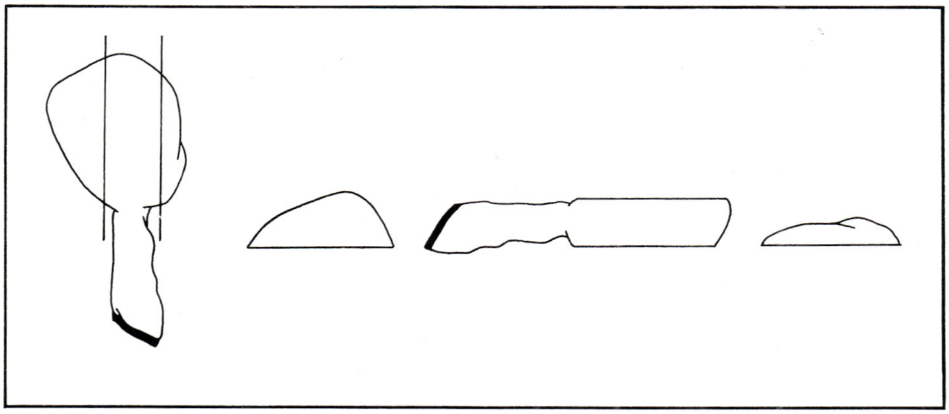

6a A pedunculated polyp with a long stalk of normal mucosa over a fibrovascular core of submucosa (▶).

6b Blocks from a pedunculated polyp. Those with slender stalks should be trimmed as shown, leaving the stalk intact. Several histological sections should then be cut through the block that contains the stalk.

7a

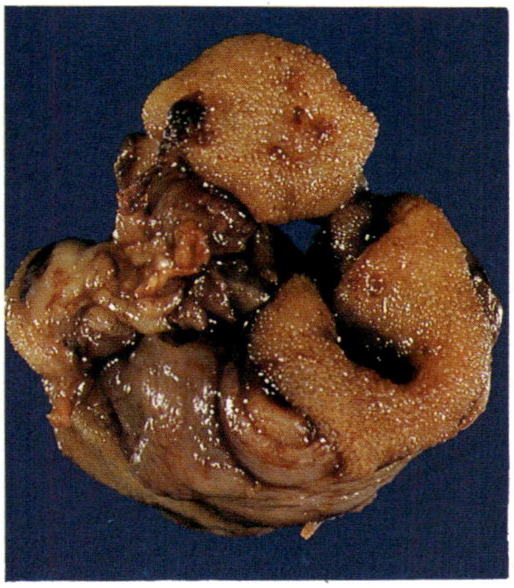

7b

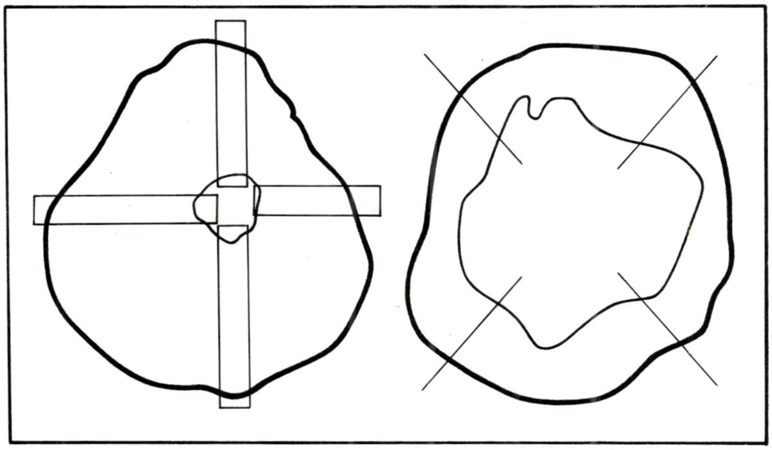

7a Ring from the excision end of the bowel taken at a colectomy operation (in this case the ring is relatively thick).

7b Dissection of rings of bowel wall. Sutures and staples must be removed before the tissue is blocked. Depending on the size of the ring, dissection can be by parallel longitudinal blocks, useful if the ring is thick, or by radial longitudinal cuts to make circumferential blocks from short rings.

Resection specimens

General

Most specimens will be received fixed or partly fixed. After measurements have been made, the way that the specimen is opened will depend on the type of resection and site of the lesion. These are given in detail below. The tissue is then pinned out onto a cork board, immersed in formalin, and left to fix fully (**8a**). When fixed it is dissected to display the full extent of the pathology and appropriate blocks are taken.

For all alimentary tract specimens, longitudinally-orientated blocks are taken, except when there is a good reason not to. Blocks from resection margins can also be longitudinal or can be circumferential around the entire margin (**8b**). Practice varies in this, but on the whole if a defined tumour mass is present, longitudinal blocks are more useful in assessing the proximity of the tumour to the excision line. This method has the advantage that the excision margin itself is seen on the microscope slides. If diffuse infiltration is suspected, circumferential blocks are more likely to demonstrate small foci of tumour near the excision margin. However, the latter method may not show the resection line itself because the tissue at the excision line either remains deep in the block or is lost when the block is trimmed.

Dissection of the lymph nodes will be required in cancer cases and specimens involved by certain other disease processes. It is usual to state in the macroscopic report the number of lymph nodes which appear to be involved by metastatic tumour, though the value of this is debatable. The stated number is often lower than the number of nodes found to be involved on microscopical examination. In such cases the macroscopical description has to be adjusted at a later date, or left as it is (since it is factually correct) and two numbers reported, at the risk of confusing the clinicians. At dissection, the record should be confined to the number of nodes found at the time, so that the number

8a

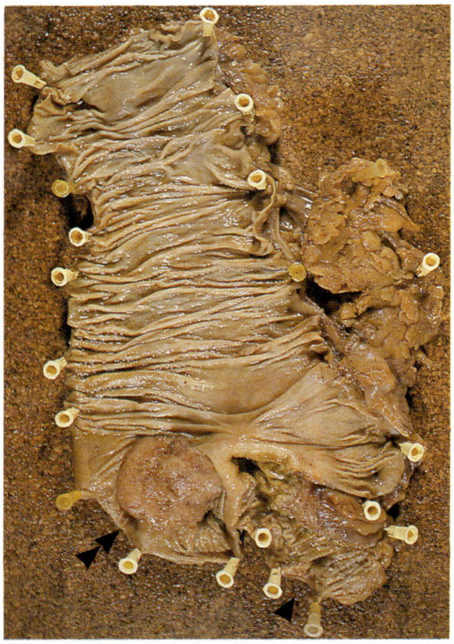

8b

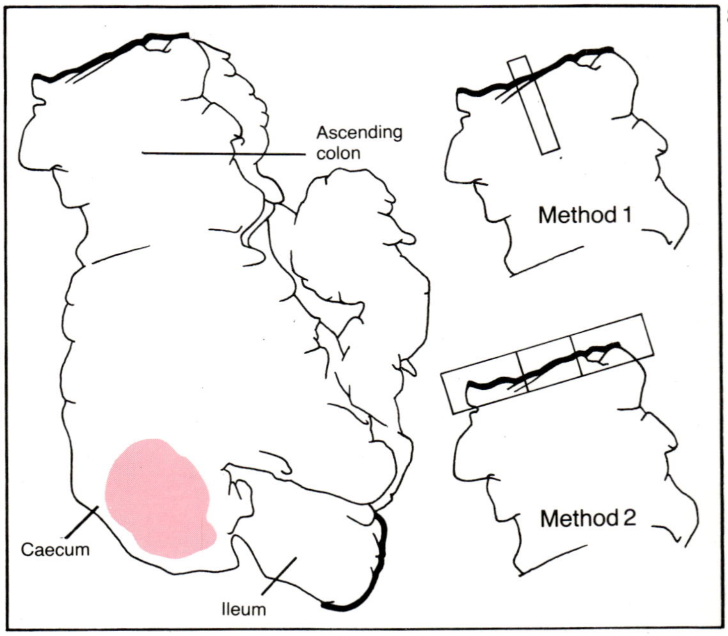

8a A right hemicolectomy specimen comprising 7 cm of terminal ileum (▶) and 23 cm of large bowel. In the caecum there is a polypoid tumour protruding into the lumen (▶▶). The specimen has been opened along the antimesenteric border and pinned out onto a cork board to fix.

8b Blocks taken from the large bowel. The resection lines of a tubular organ such as the large bowel can be sampled either by taking a block longitudinally through the excision margin in line with the nearest aspect of the lesion (Method 1); or by removing 0.5 cm of tissue at the excision margin and dividing it up to form circumferential blocks (Method 2).

of lymph node sections can be correlated with the number of nodes submitted for histology.

Dissection of lymph nodes

In most pathology departments this is done after fixation, and is usually most easily done before the rest of the specimen is dissected. The serosa of the organ or the adipose tissue of the omentum, mesentery or mesocolon is palpated for firm nodules, and slices are made through any that are found. Slices are then made at close intervals through the adipose tissue to reveal those nodes that were impalpable. Lymph nodes are seen as round or oval grey-white nodules in most cases, but may occasionally be haemorrhagic or replaced by uniform yellow adipose tissue (**9**). In practice, half (or all, if very small) of any discrete structure discovered in the mesenteric fat or serosa of the alimentary tract should be blocked.

When nodes are difficult to find, clearing of the adipose tissue from the specimen with xylene may be considered. The tissue is immersed in several times its own volume of xylene and left overnight to clear. Large specimens will need a change of xylene and a further period of immersion. It is doubtful whether the results of this technique are worth the time, effort and mess involved.

In large specimens, the sites from which the nodes are obtained and the number found at each site should be recorded. Nodes from different areas should be blocked separately.

Oesophagus

Types of specimen

Oesophagectomy is performed principally for malignancy, and very rarely for non-neoplastic conditions. The specimen will often include part of the stomach. If the malignancy is in the upper third of the oesophagus, part of the pharynx may be attached.

Initial dissection

The specimen should be palpated to establish the site and extent of malignancy. If the tumour is not circumferential, the specimen should be opened through the part of the wall which is not involved (**10a**). If it does involve the entire circumference, the oesophagus is opened along the left lateral aspect. Inferiorly, the opening cut should extend along the greater curve of the stomach if this is present (**11**). After opening, the specimen should be pinned out onto a cork board and allowed to fix fully.

Dissection of specimen

The oesophagus and attached tissues should be measured before dissection. If it is likely to be difficult to assess the completeness of the excision of a tumour, the deep, proximal and distal resection margins of the specimen should be marked with India ink. After the mucosal aspect of the lesion has been examined, several longitudinal parallel cuts should be made into it through to the serosa, to display the extent of invasion (**12**). The perioesophageal adipose tissue should be examined for lymph nodes. The sites of these

9

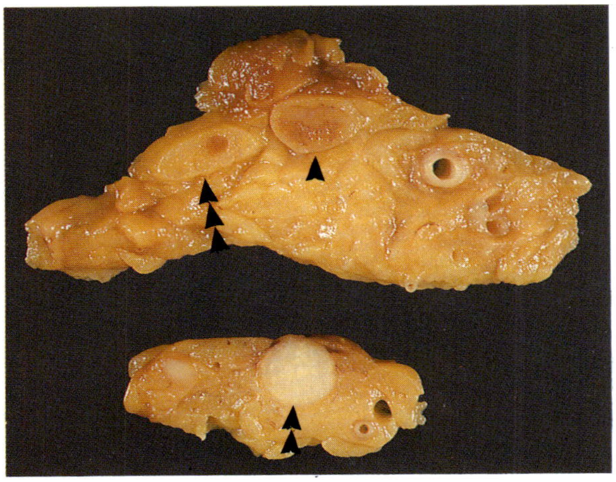

9 Lymph nodes in the adipose tissue of the mesentery. These usually appear as ovoid or round nodules with translucent pink centres (▶). When replaced by tumour the cut surface is densely white or grey (▶▶), and when replaced largely by adipose tissue they are uniformly yellow and soft (▶▶▶).

Oesophagus: Macroscopical report

Type of specimen	Partial oesophagectomy, oesophagogastrectomy, upper oesophagus with pharynx
Overall measurements	Length and circumference of the opened specimen Lengths of lesser and greater curves of stomach and/or other tissues present
Tumour	Site and size of tumour Distance of the tumour from the oesophagogastric squamocolumnar junction, and from the surgical excision ends Colour Consistency (mucoid, firm) Texture (ulcerated, granular) Contour (constricted, polypoid, dilated) Depth of penetration of the wall, and involvement of structures outside the wall such as bronchus or pericardium Cephalic and caudal spread within the submucosa (this can be very difficult to judge macroscopically)
Rest of oesophagus	Stricture, irregular white plaques, varices, dilatation
Lymph nodes	Sites and numbers

(upper, middle or lower third of oesophagus, fundus, lesser curve and greater curve of stomach) and the number found at each site should be recorded.

Blocks are taken from the resection margins, the tumour and the adjacent oesophageal wall, the uninvolved oesophagus and stomach, the squamocolumnar junction and from any other tissues present, such as diaphragm muscle, pericardium and liver (**10b**). The lymph nodes in the specimen are identified as described above (**9**).

Example 11-12

The specimen consists of a resection of lower oesophagus and fundus of stomach, received as two parts. One consists of 5.5 cm of oesophagus, and the other of 5 cm of distal oesophagus and gastric fundus measuring 4 cm along the lesser curve and 9.5 cm along the greater. The diameter of the oesophagus in both parts is 4.3 cm.

At 1.1 cm from the proximal oesophageal excision line and 6 cm from the squamocolumnar junction of the reconstituted specimen there is a partly ulcerated, polypoid, white annular tumour measuring 3.3 cm long and protruding 0.8 cm above the surface of the adjacent mucosa. The cut section shows that the tumour has penetrated the full thickness of the wall of the oesophagus and has reached the serosa.

The uninvolved oesophageal mucosa shows no significant abnormality. The gastric mucosa and wall are unremarkable. Several soft lymph nodes are identified in the serosa of the oesophagus and fundus.

Blocks

- **A** proximal oesophageal excision line × 2
- **B** lesser curve excision line × 1
- **C** tumour × 3
- **D** uninvolved oesophageal wall × 1
- **E** squamocolumnar junction × 1
- **F** uninvolved gastric wall × 2
- **G** lymph nodes from mid oesophagus × 2
- **H** lymph nodes from lower oesophagus × 4
- **J** lymph nodes from lesser curve × 2
- **K** lymph nodes from greater curve × 5

10a

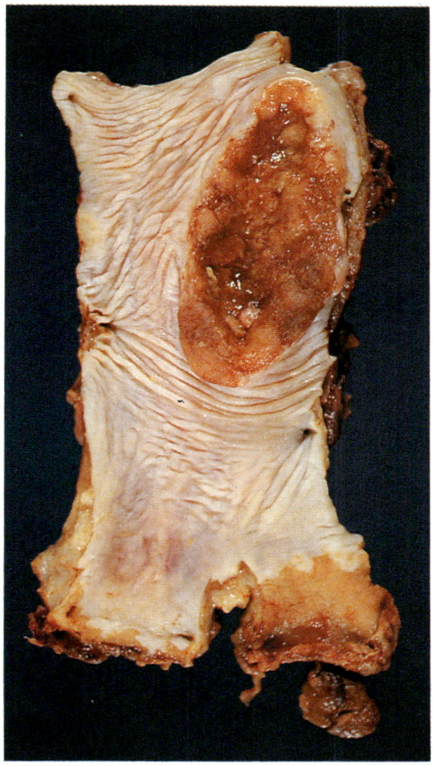

10b

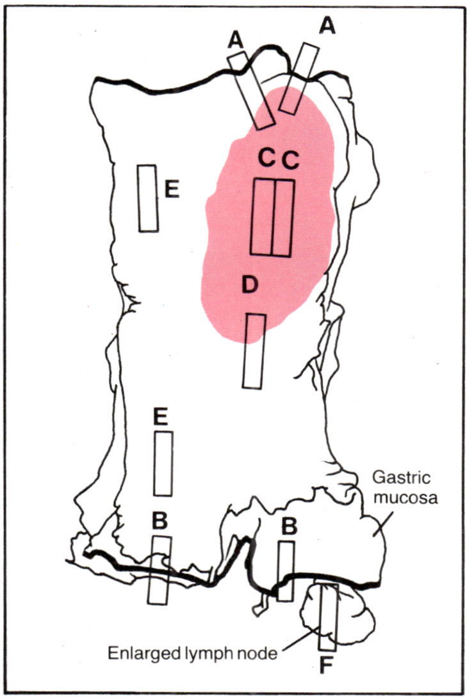

10a An oesophagectomy specimen (with a small strip of gastric mucosa at the bottom) which has been opened through the left lateral wall of the oesophagus, avoiding the carcinoma in the upper half. A block was removed for frozen section from the gastric excision line.

10b Blocks taken from an oesophagectomy specimen: proximal excision margin (**A**); gastric wall and distal excision margin (**B**); centre of tumour (**C**); tumour and adjacent oesophagus (**D**); uninvolved oesophageal wall (**E**); lymph nodes from distal half of specimen (**F**); lymph nodes from proximal half of specimen (**G**—not shown).

11

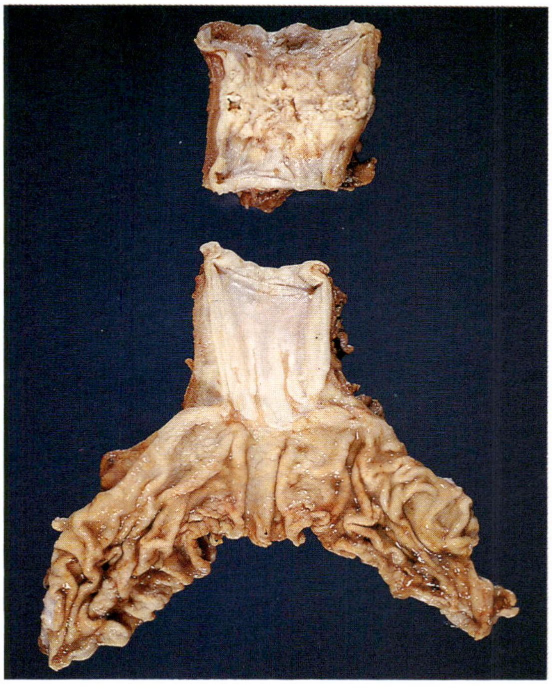

12

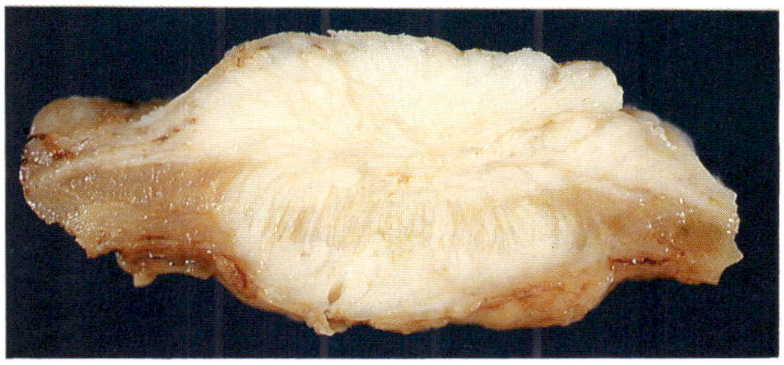

11 An oesophagectomy specimen with upper part of stomach. The middle part (5 cm) of the oesophagus was removed separately from the lower part of the specimen for surgical reasons. The oesophagus has been opened along the left lateral wall and the cut extended down the greater curve of the stomach. The smaller specimen, from the middle oesophagus, shows a circumferential invasive carcinoma.

12 Cross section through the oesophageal carcinoma in 11. The tumour has extended through the submucosa, muscularis propria and serosa into the adjacent adipose tissue.

Stomach

Types of specimen

Gastrectomy specimens from a patient with primary gastric disease may consist of a sheet of gastric wall or a partial or total gastrectomy. In addition, the stomach or parts of it may be removed as part of a more extensive procedure for disease elsewhere, such as a Whipple's operation (p 36) or an oesophagogastrectomy (p 17).

Gastrectomies are usually performed for peptic ulceration and malignant disease (**13-18**). Specimens from patients with peptic ulcers do not always include the ulcer, which may be in the duodenum. If no ulcer is found and the information on the request form is unhelpful, the clinicians should be consulted for clarification.

Initial dissection

The stomach should be opened along the greater curve (**13, 14**), unless the request form or inspection or palpation of the specimen indicates that there is a lesion on it, in which case the lesser curve should be opened. The oesophagus and duodenum, if present, should be opened in continuity with the gastric incision and pinned out for further fixation if necessary. If a large volume of adipose tissue is attached to the lesser and greater curves, the cardiac and the pyloric aspects should be marked and it should be removed and fixed separately.

Dissection of specimen

Before dissection the specimen should be measured. The serosal surface and excision ends of the specimen may be marked with India ink if a neoplasm is suspected, and any lesions present should be measured and described. Parallel longitudinal cuts should be made into them through to the serosa to assess the depth of involvement of the stomach wall (**18**).

Blocks should be taken from any focal lesions and adjacent tissue, and from the uninvolved stomach in at least two places (such as the anterior and posterior walls), as well as from the resection margins if a neoplasm or dysplasia is suspected or identified (**17b**). If there is diffuse thickening of the wall of the stomach, several blocks should be taken to look for infiltration by carcinoma. The adipose tissue attached to the lesser curve, greater curve, cardia and pylorus

Stomach: Macroscopical report	
Type of specimen	Sheet of gastric wall, partial gastrectomy, total gastrectomy, oesophagogastrectomy, part of a Whipple's operation
Other organs	Oesophagus, duodenum, pancreas, spleen
Overall measurements	Lengths of lesser and greater curves, and of oesophagus and duodenum if attached
Major lesions	
Neoplasm	Size; site; growth pattern (fungating, ulcerating, flat, diffuse); colour; consistency (friable, fibrous, soft) Extent of spread (within and through the stomach wall, into contiguous organs, proximity to excision margins)
Ulcer	Diameter; depth; site; colour; contour (stellate, round, ovoid, with raised edges); texture (debris at ulcer base, granularity, exposed large vessels, penetration of other tissues such as liver or pancreas); consistency (firm, oedematous)
Diffuse disease	Hyperplasia, inflammation, atrophy
Rest of stomach	Mucosa away from lesion; colour; texture (eroded, ulcerated, hyperplastic); contour (distorted by fibrosis, constricted)
Lymph nodes	Sites and numbers
Other organs	Weight; measurements; macroscopic lesions

(and omentum if present) should be examined for lymph nodes as described above. Nodes from these various sites should be identified and blocked separately.

Example 16-18

The specimen consists of a partial gastrectomy measuring 12 cm along the lesser curve and 15 cm along the greater curve. No oesophagus or duodenum is attached. The serosa over the upper anterior aspect of the lesser curve shows haemorrhagic discoloration. On opening the stomach, in the body on the lesser curve there is a punched-out ulcer 0.8 cm in diameter, 3.1 cm from the proximal resection margin. A small superficial erosion is also present, 2.2 cm from the proximal resection margin, adjacent to but separate from the area of ulceration. The cut section through the ulcer base shows dense, firm white tissue extending into the adjacent submucosa, muscularis propria and serosa. Around the ulcer, the mucosal folds radiate outwards and are severely thickened.

Elsewhere in the specimen, the gastric rugae are prominent, but no other focal lesion is apparent. Eight enlarged lymph nodes ranging from 0.8 to 1.5 cm in diameter are present in the adipose tissue attached to the lesser curve, and two small nodes each 0.5 cm in diameter are present on the greater curve.

Blocks

A proximal resection margin in the line of the ulcer including erosion × 1
B distal resection margin in the line of the ulcer × 1
C ulcer and surrounding tissue × 2
D body mucosa away from ulcer × 2
E antral mucosa away from ulcer × 1
F lesser curve lymph nodes × 8
G greater curve lymph nodes × 2

13

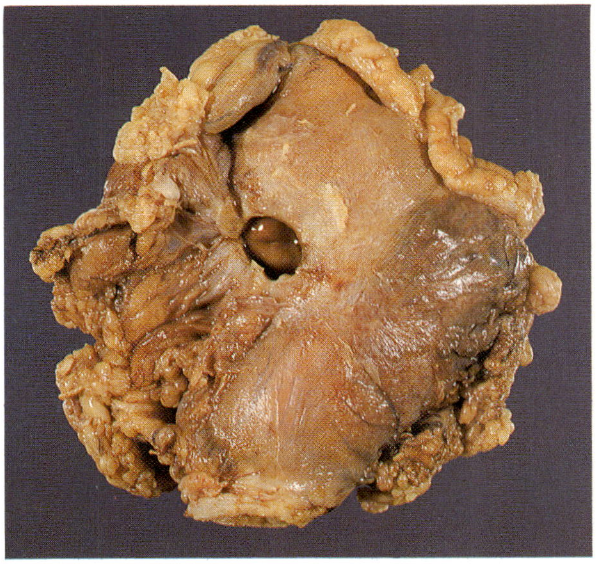

13 A partial gastrectomy specimen with attached greater and lesser curve adipose tissue. The serosal surface of the anterior gastric wall shows an area of perforation. Around this the serosa is congested and focally haemorrhagic. The adipose tissue on the lesser curve is inflamed and fibrosed in the area of the ulcer.

14

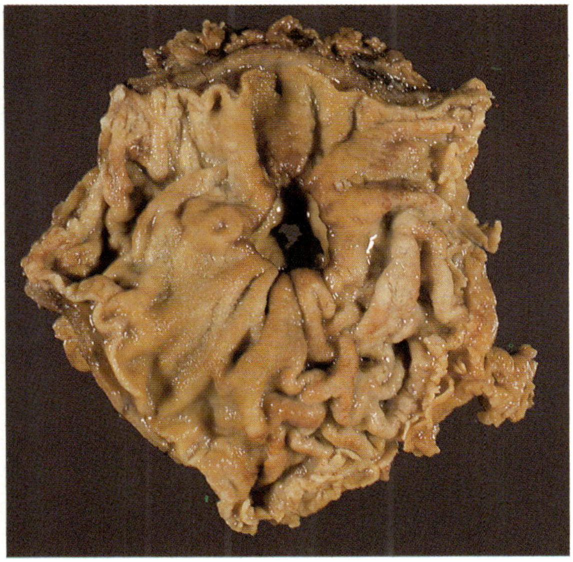

14 The stomach in 13 opened along the greater curve to show a cleanly perforated peptic ulcer in the body of the stomach on the lesser curve. The radial pattern of rugae around the ulcer has been produced by fibrosis and subsequent contraction.

15

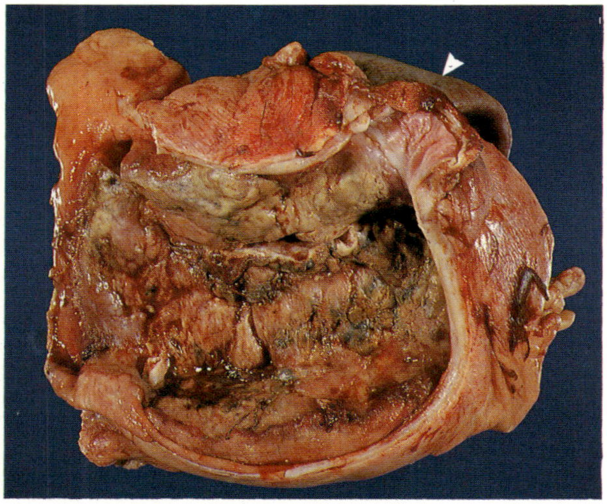

15 The fundus and body of the stomach opened along the greater curve. There is diffuse thickening of the posterior gastric wall with extensive mucosal ulceration. Microscopically this was found to be caused by invasive carcinoma. The spleen (▶) was excised as a necessary surgical manoeuvre. (The gastric antrum was also removed and sent as a separate specimen.)

16

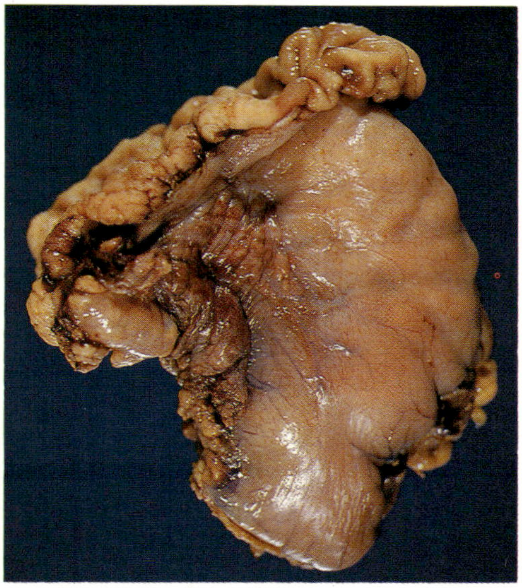

16 A partial gastrectomy specimen showing haemorrhagic discoloration over the upper anterior aspect of the lesser curve.

17a Specimen 16 opened along the greater curve to reveal a punched-out ulcer and a small erosion on the lesser curve (▶).

17a

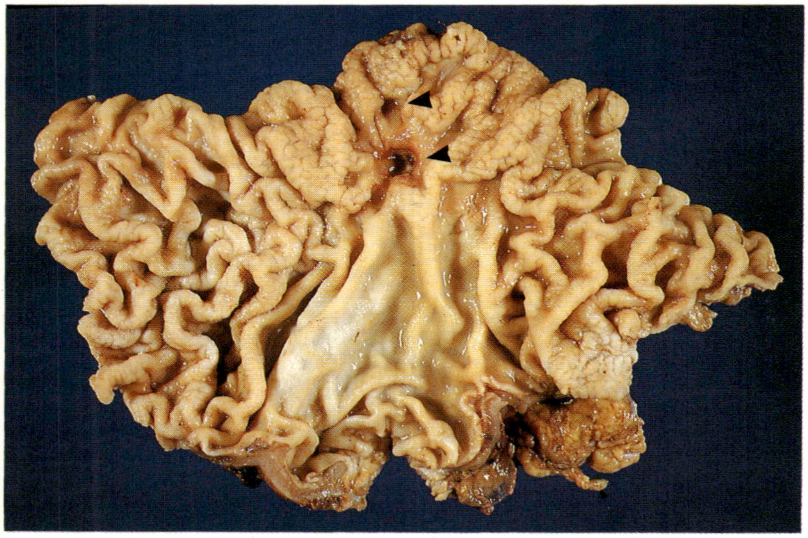

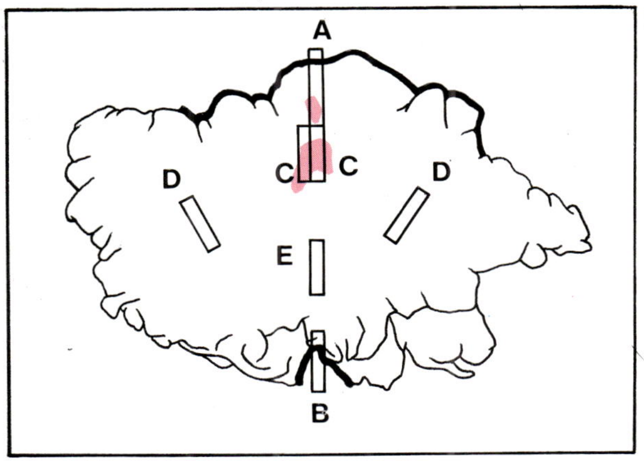

17b

17b Blocks taken from a partial gastrectomy specimen with a focal lesion: proximal excision margin in the line of the ulcer including erosion (**A**); distal excision margin (**B**); ulcer and surrounding tissue (**C**); body mucosa away from ulcer (**D**); antral mucosa away from ulcer (**E**); lesser curve lymph nodes (**F**—not shown); greater curve lymph nodes (**G**—not shown).

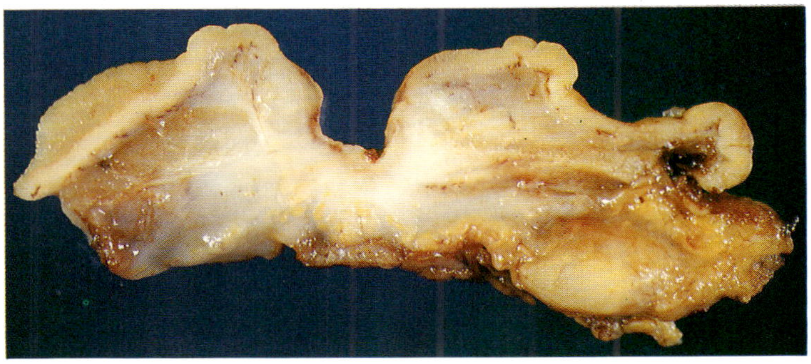

18

18 A longitudinal slice through the ulcer in 17.

Appendix and Meckel's Diverticulum

Type of specimen

The appendix is one of the commonest histological specimens. The whole organ is always removed, with or without the mesoappendix. The purpose of pathological examination in almost all cases is to establish whether appendicitis is present, and if so what has caused it. Appendicitis is usually idiopathic, but occasionally there will be macroscopical evidence of a carcinoid tumour, carcinoma, mucocele (**19**), stricture (**20**) or other aetiological agent.

A specimen of a Meckel's diverticulum (**21**) includes a short length of ileum on either side of the diverticulum so that its neck, where ectopic acid-secreting gastric mucosa is most commonly found, can be removed entirely.

Dissection of specimen

This should be done after fixation. The appendix is measured and the serosa examined for congestion or a fibrinous or purulent exudate (**22**) (this may, of course, be secondary to inflammation outside the appendix, such as a tubal or ovarian lesion or a pericolic abscess from any cause). The specimen should be sliced transversely at 0.5 cm intervals or less (**23**), and the luminal contents, dilatation, distortion or other macroscopic abnormality should be described. If the mesoappendix is attached this will keep the sections in sequence. The tip should be cut in half longitudinally (**23, 24**).

A Meckel's diverticulum can be treated in the same way as an appendix, or both the attached ileum and the diverticulum can be opened in a T-shape (**21b**). Blocks should be taken from different sites along the diverticulum, but especially from around the mouth, and identified separately. The contralateral ileal wall should be examined histologically for ulceration, erosion or inflammation.

Appendix and Meckel's diverticulum: Macroscopical report

Measurements	Length and maximum diameter Length of small bowel, if present
Description	
Serosa	Congested, covered by fibrinous exudate, haemorrhage, involvement by tumour
Cut surface of wall	Fibrosed, distorted, perforated, constricted
Mucosa and luminal contents	Faecolith; identifiable food particles such as grape pips; pus

Example 22-24

The specimen consists of an appendix measuring 7.5 cm in length and 0.9 cm in maximum diameter. The serosa is congested and covered by a patchy fibrinopurulent exudate. No obvious perforation is evident in the wall. The lumen contains a small amount of pus. No faecoliths are present.

Blocks × 3

19

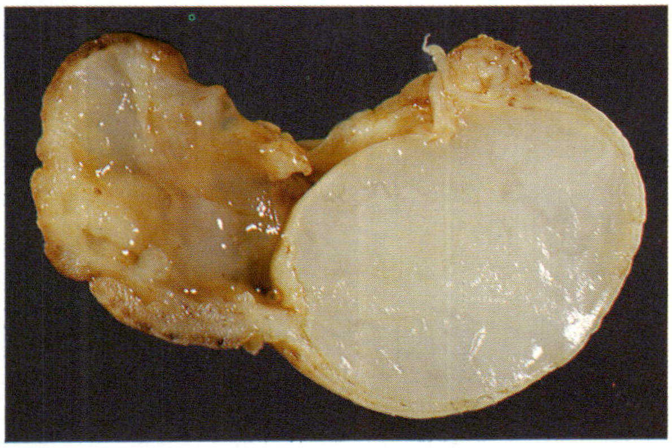

19 Mucocele of the appendix. There has been distention of the appendix lumen near the tip by the tumour, which is producing thick, clear mucus.

20

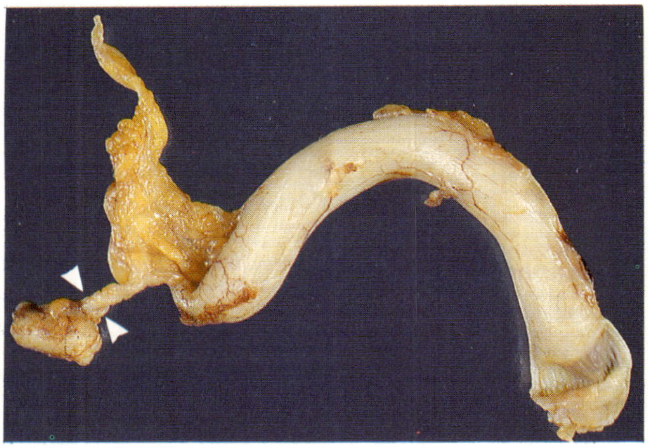

20 An appendix showing fibrosis of the tip, which is connected to the rest of the organ by a tough fibrous band (▶).

21a

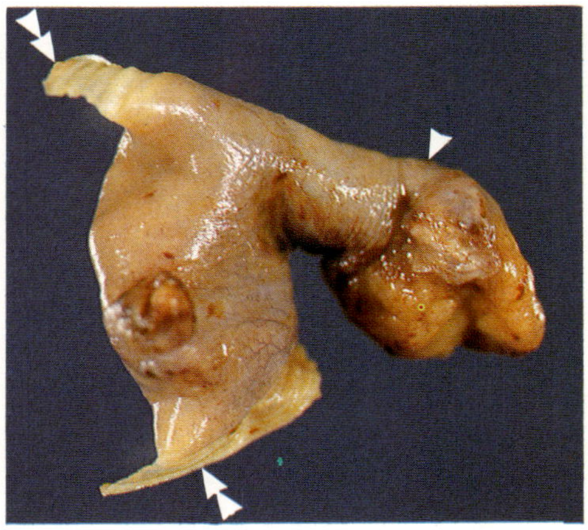

21a A Meckel's diverticulum (▶) removed with a small segment of attached ileal wall. Clamp marks are visible at the proximal and distal ileal resection margins (▶▶).

21b Blocks taken from a Meckel's diverticulum specimen: tip of diverticulum (**A**); mouth of diverticulum (**B**); ileum (**C**).

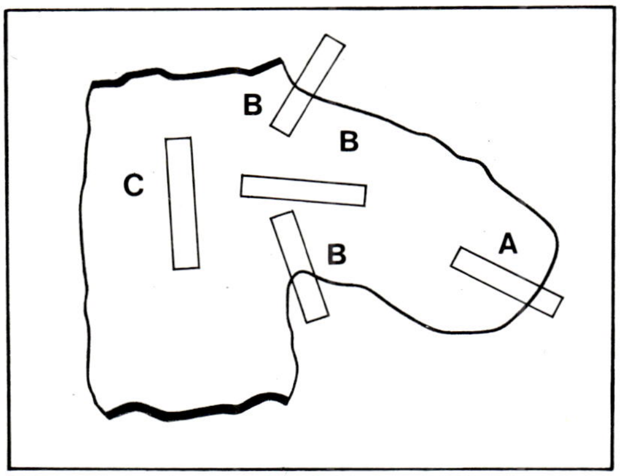

21b

22 Acute purulent appendicitis with overlying peritonitis. The serosa of the appendix is severely congested and covered by a patchy fibrinopurulent exudate.

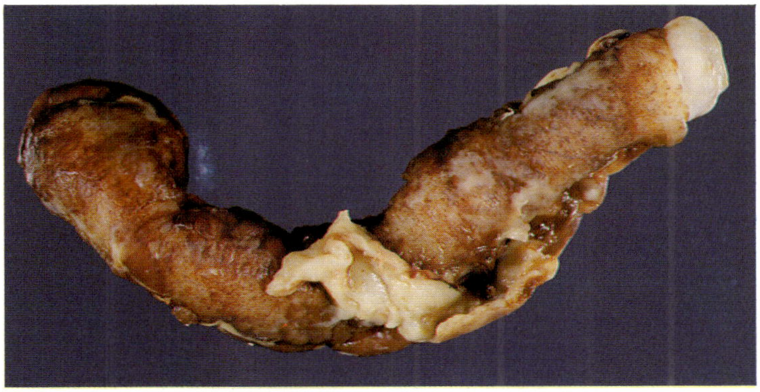

22

23 Transverse parallel cuts through 22 up to the tip, which is bisected longitudinally.

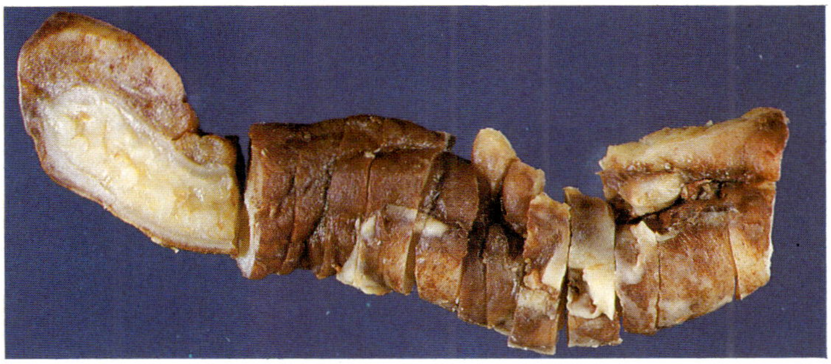

23

24 Blocks taken from appendix 22. Three or four blocks of an appendix are usually taken depending on its length and the pathology found. These include a longitudinal section of the tip.

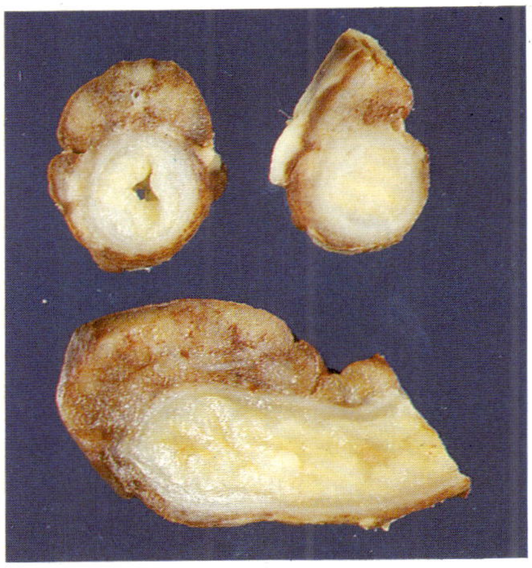

24

25

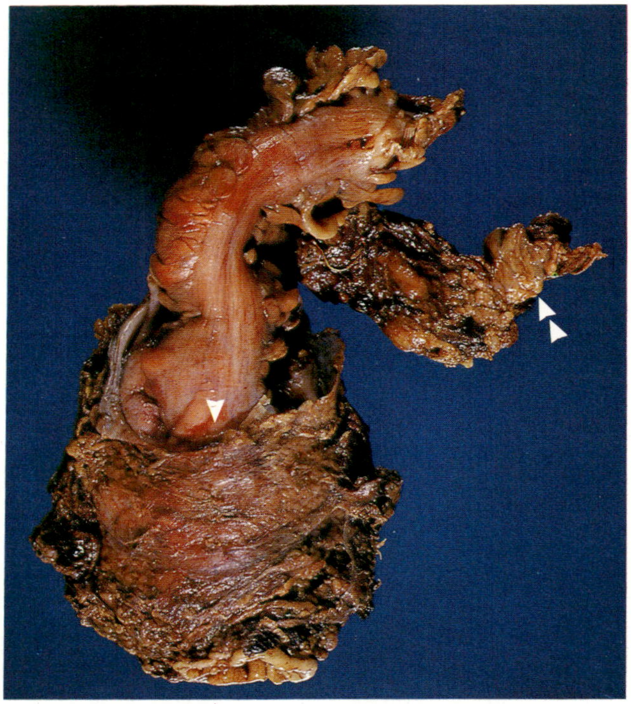

25 Orientation of a combined anteroposterior resection of the rectum. The anterior surface shows the peritoneal reflection (▶). The lower sigmoid mesocolon and vascular tie are also shown (▶▶).

26

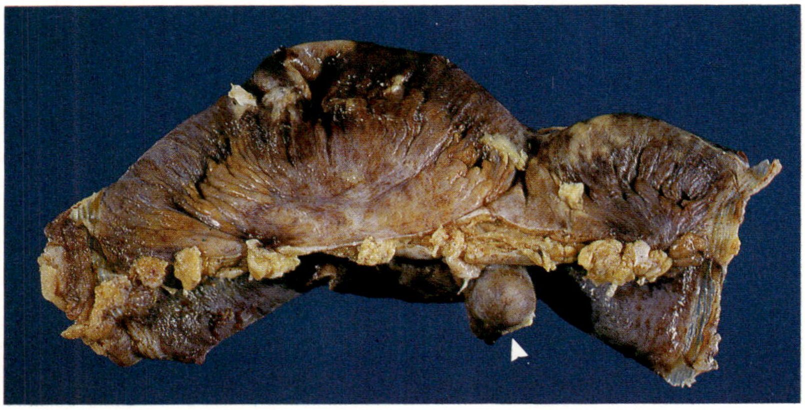

26 A length of small bowel containing a Meckel's diverticulum (▶). The serosal surface is severely congested and shows a patchy purulent exudate.

27

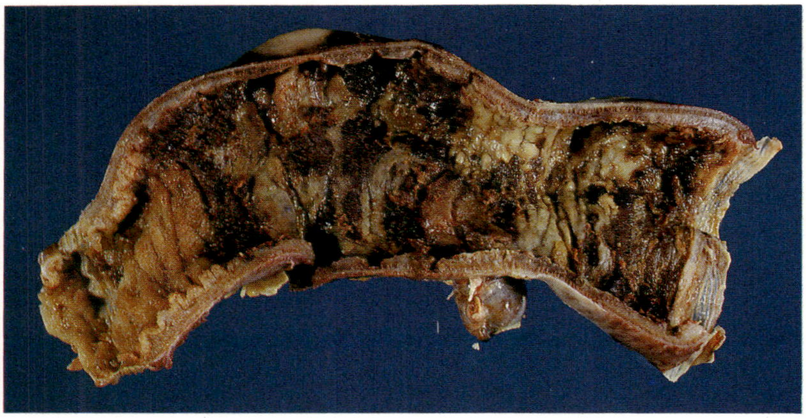

27 Specimen 26 opened along the antimesenteric border. There is extensive shallow ulceration of the mucosal surface and the bowel wall is thinner than normal. The 4 cm of bowel adjacent to the distal resection margin appears normal. On microscopic examination ischaemic enteritis was identified. The Meckel's diverticulum in the specimen is treated as in **21b**.

Small and Large Bowel

Types of specimen

Specimens of small bowel include lengths of bowel excised because of strangulation, ischaemia, diverticular disease, duplications and, rarely, neoplasia. Large bowel excision specimens include appendicectomy, submucosal resection of villous adenomas, colectomy, enterocolectomy, proctocolectomy and panproctocolectomy specimens. The last-named operation involves removal of perianal skin, anus, large bowel and appendix, and terminal ileum by a combined abdominal-perineal approach. Appendicectomy and Meckel's diverticulectomy specimens are dealt with separately above.

Initial Dissection

Specimens of bowel may have other organs or tissues attached, such as vagina, uterus, bladder or coccyx, and these should be identified at the initial dissection. The bowel should be palpated to establish the site and extent of any focal lesions. Rectal specimens can be orientated by the position of the peritoneal reflection (**25**). They should be opened anteriorly if possible, avoiding focal, non-circumferential lesions. Other lengths of bowel are opened along the antimesenteric or equivalent border (**26, 27**), but if there are adherent viscera or non-circumferential lesions, the cut should if possible avoid these (**28, 29**). Bowel resected for diverticular disease is often very resilient and should be treated differently (p 26).

After opening the bowel, faecal material in the lumen should be washed away with a gentle stream of cold water; the use of a jet of water can create fine spray and should be avoided. There is no good evidence that water used briefly for washing is detrimental to the specimen. If formalin solution is used instead (as preferred in some departments), great care must be taken to avoid splashes and inhalation of fumes.

If the specimen has been received fresh or partially fixed, it should be pinned out after opening and left to fix fully. Specimens received completely fixed can sometimes be opened and pinned out, but if there is stenosis or fibrous thickening this may cause cracking and distortion of the viscus. In some departments it is standard practice to fix the bowel by filling it with formalin and tying both ends. This is effective, but trying to force formalin into a constricted lumen with a syringe is dangerous and should not be considered.

Dissection of specimen

The method of dissection of the specimen will vary with different pathology. In specimens removed for malignant tumours and various inflammatory conditions, especially Crohn's disease and ulcerative colitis, the lymph nodes may be dissected first, as described on p 15. Care must be taken not to distort the deep resection margin in the area of a tumour. In tumour cases the node or group of nodes found in the most proximal part of the mesentery/mesocolon or around the vascular pedicle should be identified separately (**25**).

Nodes from different parts of the bowel (caecum, ascending, transverse, descending and sigmoid colon and rectum) should be labelled separately. In a panproctocolectomy specimen removed because of longstanding ulcerative colitis with dysplasia, invasive malignancy can sometimes be difficult to identify macroscopically. The bowel can be divided into notional 20 cm lengths and the lymph nodes in each stretch given an identifying number or letter, so that if metastatic tumour is found in any of the nodes, the specimen can then easily be re-examined to search for the primary tumour.

The mucosal surface should be carefully examined. Focal lesions such as inflammatory stenoses and tumours should be measured and described; the number, sites and sizes of polyps should be recorded; and the extent and pattern of ulceration should be noted. Incisions into the bowel wall to examine and take blocks from focal lesions, areas of ulceration and other pathology are usually made longitudinally, in the direction of the bowel (**30**). Incisions into the mesentery/mesocolon should be made similarly, parallel to the adjacent bowel. Examination of blocks from the proximal and distal excision margins should be undertaken if Crohn's disease, ischaemic colitis or a malignant tumour is present. This is also done in uncomplicated ulcerative colitis, but is probably of less importance. Blocks should also be taken from the deep resection margins below a malignant tumour (**28b**).

Where a tumour involves the anterior rectal wall, cuts made through it to assess the depth of invasion can be continued into the female genital organs if present, and suitable blocks taken. The coccyx is often removed at operation not because it is involved by tumour but as a necessary manoeuvre during surgery. It should be sectioned transversely with a band saw and decalcified for blocks. Occasionally, an unsuspected glomus tumour may be found within it.

When there is diverticular disease, especially of the sigmoid colon, it is often very difficult to open and pin out the specimen (**31**). If this is so, the bowel is opened longitudinally and emptied of contents to help the diffusion of formalin, but should otherwise be fixed intact. It is then sliced transversely at 0.5-1 cm intervals, leaving the mesentery to hold the sections in sequence (**32**). Diverticula are readily displayed by this method and suitable sections can be trimmed for blocks. Areas of serosal inflammation, perforation and fistula formation should be blocked first.

Local resections for carcinoma (**33a**) and submucosal resections of polyps, usually villous adenomas of the rectum, provide a specimen which consists of a partial or full-thickness sheet of bowel wall. These should be measured and the diameter and height of the lesion recorded. The excision margins should be painted with India ink before blocks are taken. Blocks should be taken from all around the specimen at right angles to the resection lines (**33b**). Numerous blocks should be examined, especially from

Bowel resection: Macroscopical report

Type of specimen	A length of small bowel or colon, a sheet of submucosa, colectomy, enterocolectomy (small intestine and colon), proctocolectomy (colon and rectum), panproctocolectomy
Measurements	Length of the component parts, starting proximally: ileum, appendix, caecum/colon/rectum, anus
Description	
Diffuse disease	*Mucosa* Colour; texture (ulcerated, granular, polypoid, cobblestone, fissured); consistency (firm, rubbery, friable, boggy) *Wall* Appearance of cut surface (thickened, fibrosed, distorted, stenosed) *Serosa* Congested, haemorrhagic, covered by fibrinous exudate *General* Extent of abnormality; proximity to excision ends; condition of the mesentery
Focal disease	
Tumour	*Appearance* Site; size; growth pattern (circumferential, polypoid, ulcerated, stenosing) *Spread* Local spread into and through bowel wall; proximity to excision margins, relation to the anorectal junction if present *General* Appearance of bowel away from tumour (polyps, colitis, ulceration)
Stenosis	*Appearance* Site; length and diameter of lumen and of wall of involved bowel *General* Appearance; diameter and length of bowel proximal and distal to stenosis; appearance of blood vessels (atheromatous, thrombosed, congested, blocked by embolus)
Diverticular disease	*Appearance* Site; length and diameter of involved bowel; estimate of number of diverticula; range of sizes; presence of faecaliths, inflammation, perforation, fistula formation *General* Other pathology present, such as polyps, ulceration
Other tissues	Number of lymph nodes found in the specimen or its parts

areas where there is uncertainty about the completeness of excision. The blocks should include the deep as well as the lateral resection margins.

Example 34-36

The proctocolectomy specimen comprises 8.1 cm of terminal ileum and 94 cm of large bowel. An appendix 8.5 cm long and 0.8 cm in diameter is attached to the caecum. Centred at a point 8 cm from the distal resection line there is a circumferential ulcerated, stenosing tumour 2.5 cm wide and 7.8 cm long. The cut section shows that this extends through the full thickness of the rectal wall into the adjacent adipose tissue and is 0.4 cm from the deep excision margin. The mucosa and proximal to the tumour as far as the hepatic flexure, has lost the normal haustral pattern and is flattened.

The descending and upper sigmoid colon show several confluent, sessile, plaque-like projections. The transverse and ascending colon, caecum and small bowel appear normal. In the area of the tumour 13 lymph nodes are found, and 23 further nodes are present elsewhere in the specimen.

Blocks

A	distal excision line × 1
B	dentate line × 1
C	tumour × 3
D	tumour and deep excision margin × 1
E	uninvolved upper rectum × 1
F	sigmoid colon × 3
G	descending colon × 2
H	splenic flexure × 2
J	transverse colon × 2
K	hepatic flexure × 2
L	ascending colon × 2
M	caecum × 2
N	appendix × 3
P	ileum × 1
R	node from distal vascular tie × 1
S	nodes from rectum × 5
T-W	nodes from each 20 cm length of large bowel, from sigmoid colon to caecum.

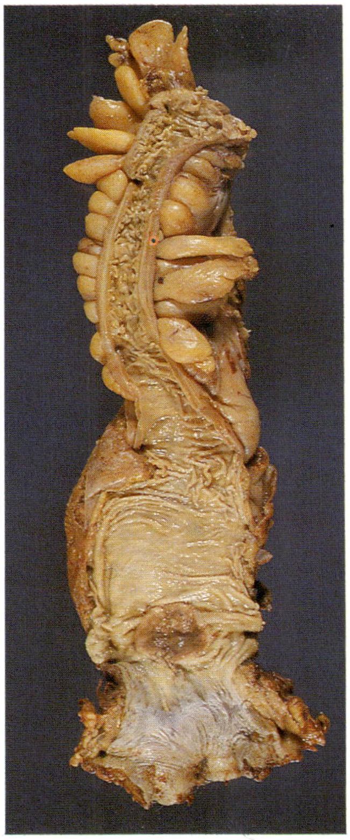

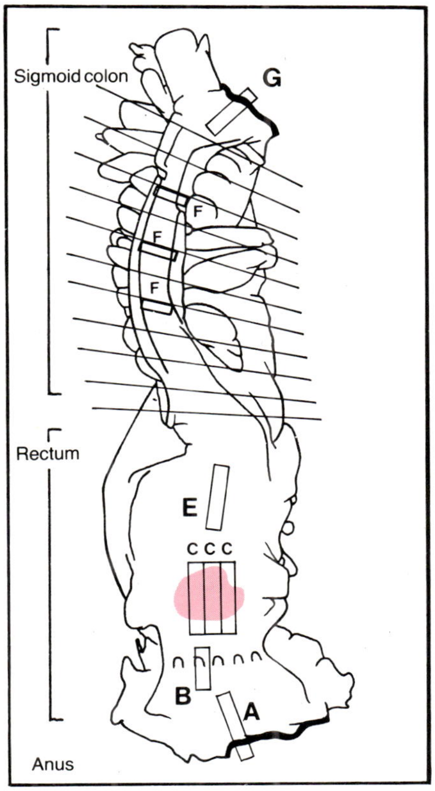

28a

28b

28a A combined abdominoperineal resection for rectal carcinoma. The specimen consists of perianal skin, anus, rectum and lower sigmoid colon. The sigmoid colon has been opened along the antimesenteric border, and the cut has then been taken down the left lateral border of the rectum to avoid the ulcerated carcinoma on the anterior wall. The sigmoid colon shows diverticular disease.

28b Blocks taken from an abdominoperineal resection specimen. If diverticular disease is present in the sigmoid colon, this part of the bowel is sectioned transversely and transverse blocks are taken (p.11). Anus and anal excision margin (**A**); dentate line (**B**); tumour (**C**); tumour and deep excision margin (**D**—not shown); uninvolved upper rectum (**E**); sigmoid colon plus diverticula (**F**); proximal excision margin (**G**); apical lymph node of sigmoid mesentery (**H**—not shown); sigmoid colon lymph nodes (**J**—not shown); rectal lymph nodes (**K**—not shown).

29

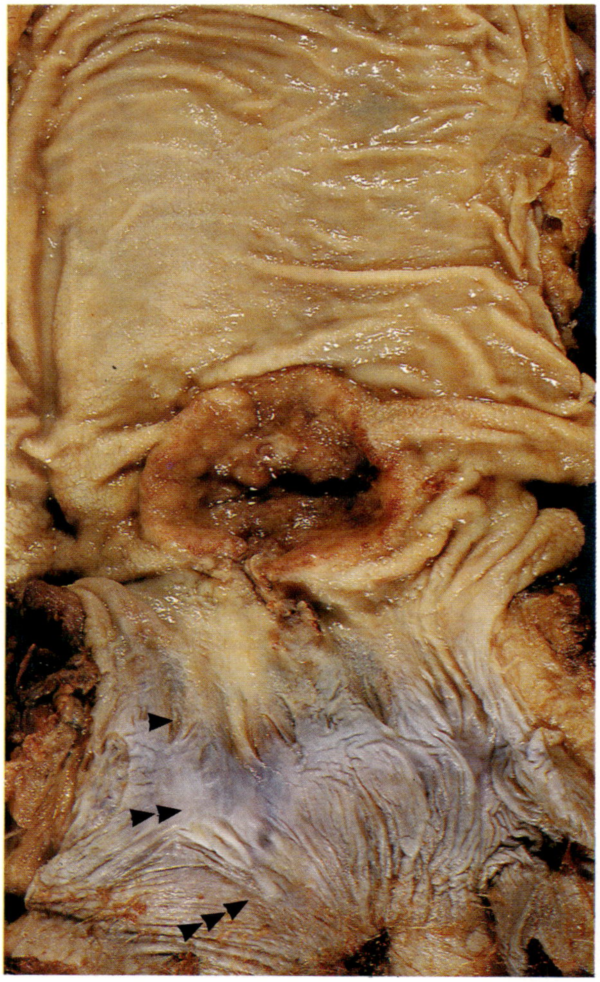

29 A detail of 28a. The raised, rolled edges of the ulcerated tumour can be seen in the lower rectum near the dentate line (▶). The pale grey mucosa of the anal canal (▶▶) and the perianal skin (▶▶▶) appear normal.

30 A longitudinal cross section of 28 showing the carcinoma. The dense white tumour tissue extends through the full thickness of the rectal wall and the adjacent fat.

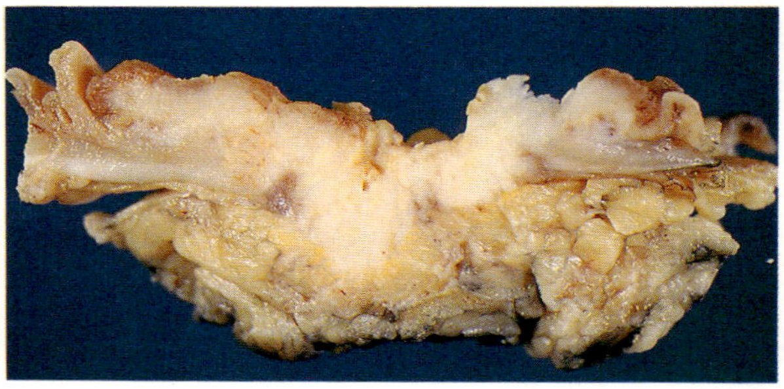

30

31

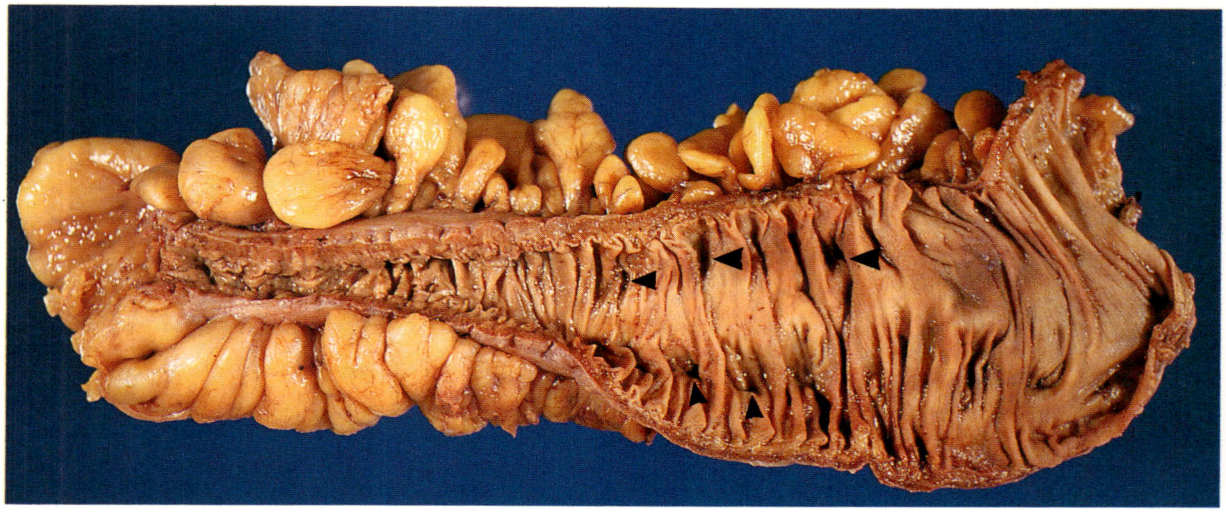

31 A sigmoid colectomy specimen with diverticular disease. The left half (proximal aspect) of the specimen was difficult to open because of the muscular hypertrophy. Ostia of diverticula can be seen in two rows near the centre of the specimen (▶).

32 A transverse cross section from 31. Muscular hypertrophy is apparent and false diverticula can be seen protruding into the pericolic adipose tissue (▶).

32

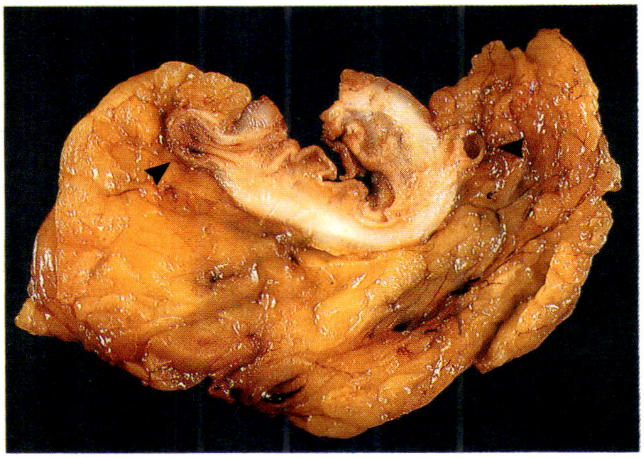

33a A full-thickness piece of bowel wall with adherent serosal adipose tissue. The mucosal surface shows a slightly raised, focally ulcerated plaque-like tumour.

33a

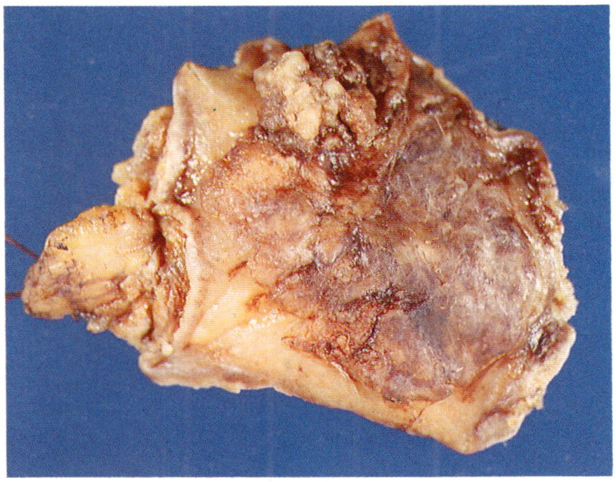

33b Blocks taken from a local resection for colonic carcinoma. Blocks should be taken radially through the lateral excision margins (**A**) and from the tumour, with underlying tissues and deep resection margin, at its centre (**B**). Any lymph nodes present are also taken for histology (**C**).

33b

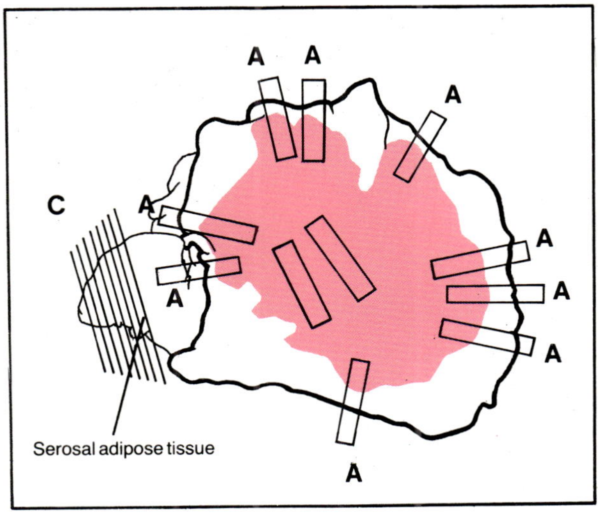

34

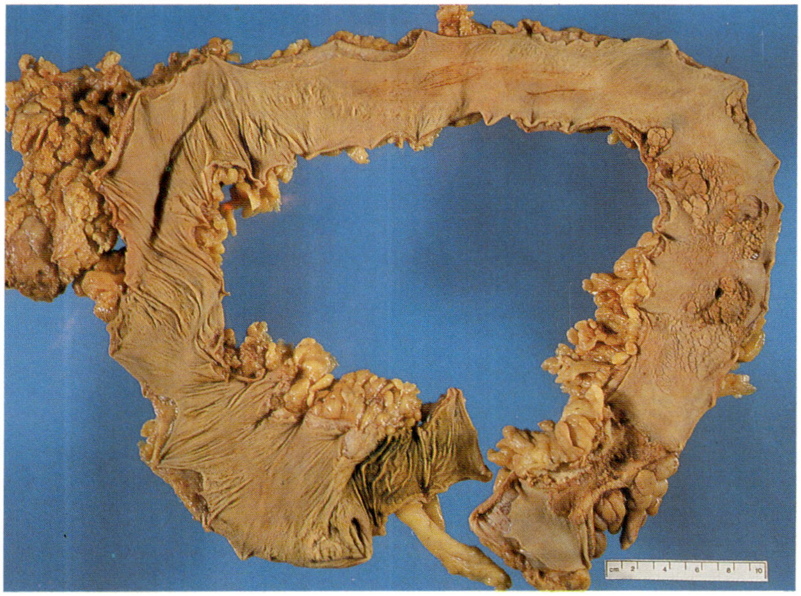

34 A proctocolectomy specimen from a patient with longstanding ulcerative colitis. There is an ulcerated annular carcinoma of the rectum and, separately, a collection of sessile polypoid projections in the left side of the colon. The mucosa distal to the hepatic flexure is flattened, typical of chronic ulcerative colitis.

35

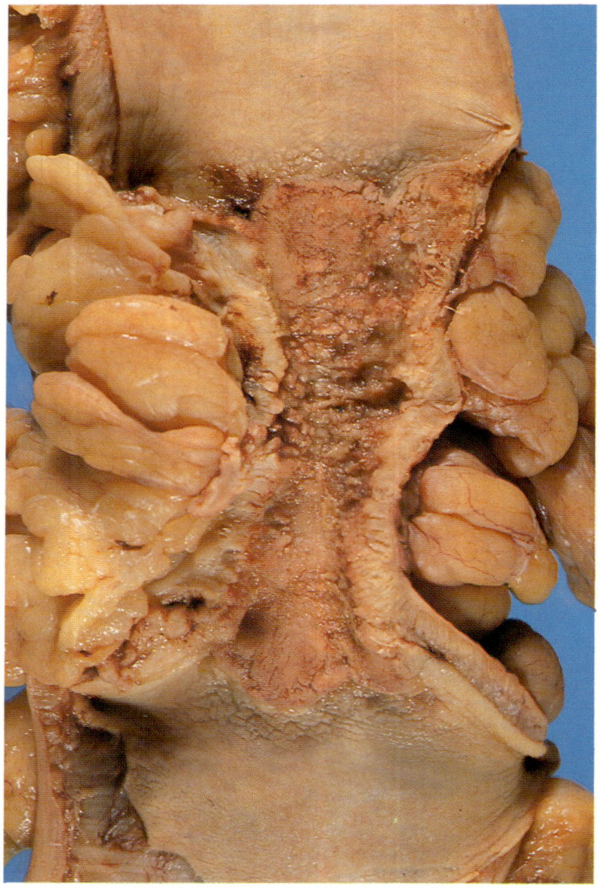

36

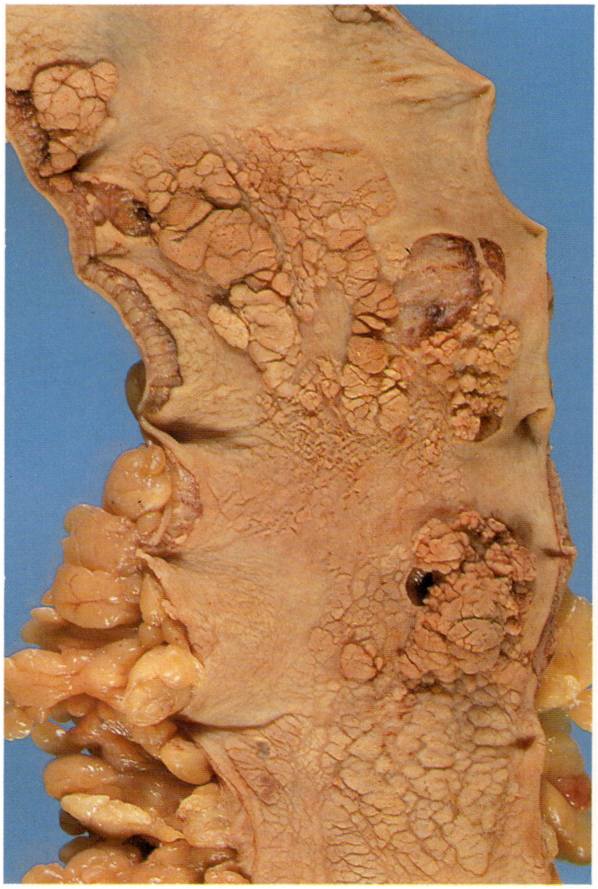

35 A detail of 34 showing the rectal carcinoma.

36 A detail of 34. On microscopic examination, the lesions in the descending colon were found to be areas of high-grade dysplasia.

CHAPTER 2
LIVER, GALL BLADDER AND PANCREAS

Liver

Small specimens

Cores of liver parenchyma are taken by Tru-cut or similar biopsy needles for the investigation of diffuse liver disease and for the diagnosis of focal deposits such as metastatic carcinoma. Wedge biopsies from the liver may be taken at laparotomy for similar reasons. In both cases, the specimen should be measured and described simply (e.g. 'A core (or wedge) of brown tissue measuring . . . all embedded'). Needle cores of tissue are embedded whole, and wedges can be cut at right angles to the capsule and the resulting slices embedded cut side down.

Large specimens

Partial hepatectomy and hemihepatectomy are performed for traumatic rupture, benign conditions such as hydatid disease of the liver and for tumours like hepatoma, if they are localized to one lobe. Metastatic carcinoma confined to one lobe is also sometimes suitable for such treatment.

Dissection of specimen

Surgery for hepatic trauma may provide several irregular pieces of liver. Their aggregate weight and range of sizes should be recorded. Photography is recommended in forensic cases.

With intact partial hepatectomy specimens, the tissue is weighed and the maximum dimensions are recorded. If neoplastic disease is suspected and may be close to the excision lines, these lines should be marked with India ink. When large specimens are received, a slice or series of slices should be made through the liver to help diffusion of formalin through the tissue. The gall bladder and large bile ducts, if present, should be opened longitudinally with fine scissors but left attached to the main specimen.

When fully fixed, a series of close parallel cuts are made through the tissue. If the liver is fragmented, the cuts are made at right angles

Liver: Macroscopical report	
Type of specimen	Needle biopsy, wedge biopsy, irregular pieces of liver, partial hepatectomy, hemihepatectomy, left lobe of liver Other tissues attached (biliary system, lymph nodes)
Measurements	Weight, if larger than needle or wedge biopsy Maximum dimensions if intact, aggregate size if fragmented
Description	
Focal lesions	Type (solitary nodule, smooth walled cyst, haematoma, tumour mass); colour; number; size or range of sizes (diameters if spherical); contour (well-defined, irregular, indistinct); consistency (firm, friable, gritty, mucoid); relation with other tissues, such as biliary system, hepatic capsule and with resection margin
Rest of liver	Congested, diffusely micronodular/macronodular, greasy and yellow, green
Other tissues	Appearance of gall bladder; dilatation or stricture of biliary system; presence of gallstones

to the capsule or in any direction if the capsule is not apparent. For intact specimens, the cuts are made sagittally (**37-39**) or at right angles to the hepatic excision margin.

Any focal or discrete abnormalities should be described and measured. Blocks are taken from these from the junction with the adjacent parenchyma, the biliary system and from the closest capsular and excision margins in cases of neoplastic disease. The uninvolved liver should also be sampled to look for pre-existing disease, microscopic tumour deposits and other conditions (**38b, 39b**).

Example 37-39

The partial hepatectomy specimen consists of the right lobe of the liver, which measures 10 × 13 × 8 cm. The attached gall bladder measures 6 × 3.5 × 4 cm and lies adjacent to the medial resection margin. In the liver there is a large, circumscribed, spherical tumour mass 8.3 cm in diameter. Its cut surface soft, variegated green and yellow tissue which extends up to, but not into, the hepatic capsule. There is no evidence of invasion into the surrounding liver parenchyma, and the resection margin appears to be tumour-free. The uninvolved liver shows micronodular cirrhosis. The gall bladder and biliary system on the specimen appear normal, and there are no gallstones. A single lymph node 1.1 cm in maximum dimension is present near the cystic duct. Its cut surface has a uniform tan-coloured appearance.

Blocks

A	centre of tumour × 2
B	tumour and hepatic capsule × 3
C	tumour and adjacent liver × 1
D	liver away from tumour × 1
E	hepatic excision margin × 4
F	gall bladder × 1
G	cystic duct lymph node × 1

37

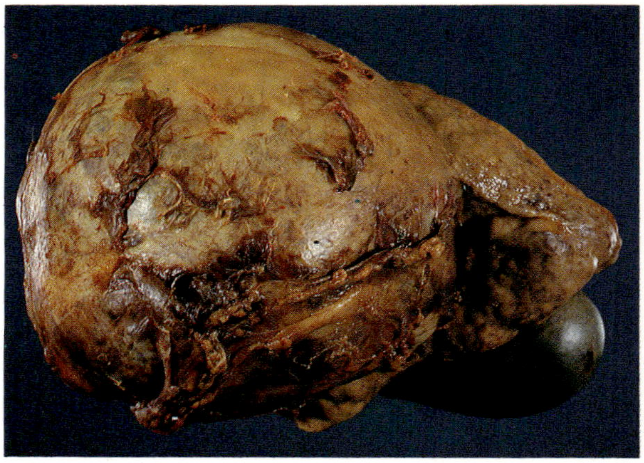

37 The lateral capsular aspect of a liver (right lobe) resected for hepatocellular carcinoma. The capsule is intact and there is no tumour on the surface of the specimen.

38a

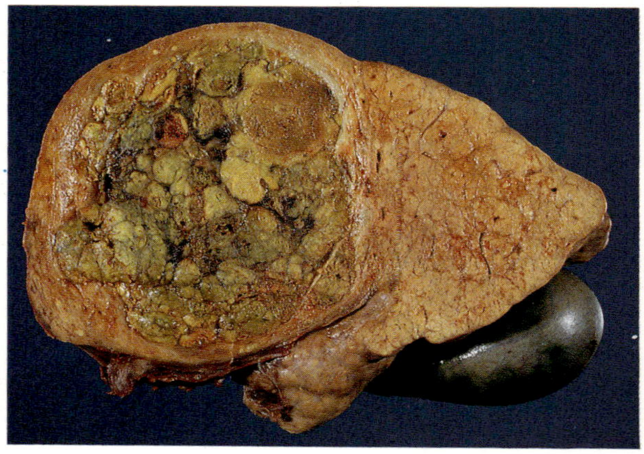

38a The cut surface of 37, a sagittal slice through the hepatocellular carcinoma. The non-neoplastic liver on the right shows micronodular cirrhosis.

38b

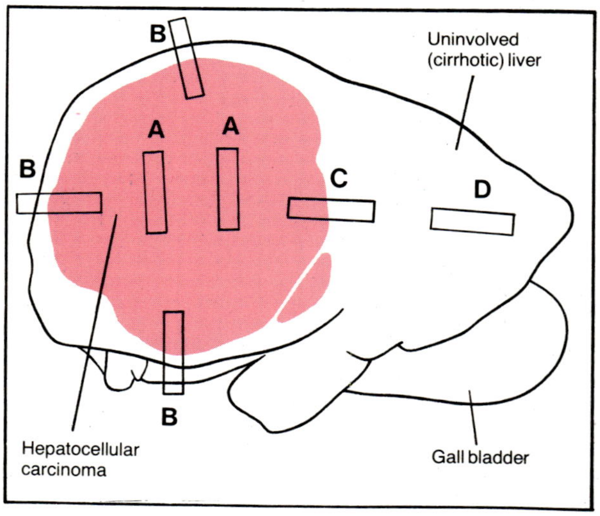

38b Blocks taken from a tumour and surrounding liver in a partial hepatectomy specimen, Part 1 (for Part 2, see **39b**): centre of tumour (**A**); tumour and hepatic capsule (**B**); tumour and adjacent liver (**C**); liver away from tumour (**D**).

39a

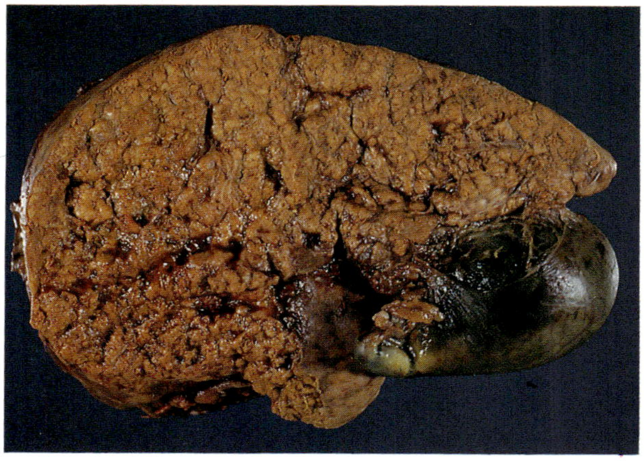

39a The resection margin of 37. The liver shows cirrhosis but no evidence of carcinoma in this area. The cystic duct lymph node is enlarged.

39b

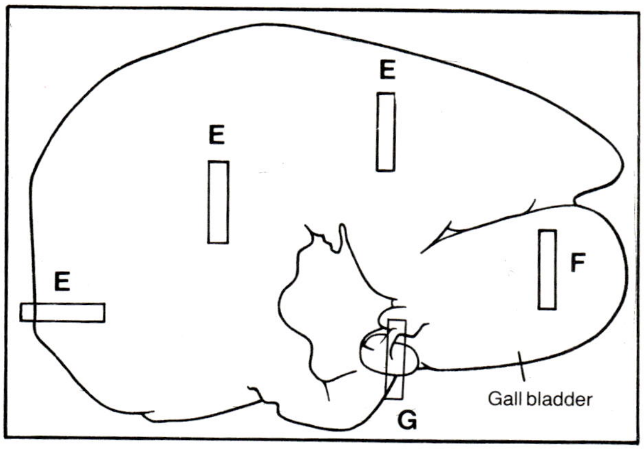

39b Blocks taken from the medial aspect of a partial hepatectomy specimen and gall bladder, Part 2: hepatic excision margin (**E**); gall bladder (**F**); cystic duct lymph node (**G**).

Gall bladder

The gall bladder may be removed for cholecystitis (with or without cholelithiasis) and rarely for carcinoma. It is often opened by the surgeon in theatre. If so, the gallstones may be removed before the specimen is sent to the laboratory.

Dissection of specimen

If the gall bladder is received intact, it is measured and opened longitudinally through the cystic duct (**40, 41**). The appearance of the contents is recorded. Thick, clear mucus (mucocele of the gall bladder) indicates that the outflow is obstructed, and the cystic duct should be examined for fibrous stricture or impacted calculi.

Calculi range from large, ovoid, smooth-surfaced cholesterol stones to tiny, gritty black pigment stones. Cholesterol stones are usually solitary. Polyhedral stones (**41**) are common; the flat surfaces or 'facets' develop between calculi as they form, and are not the result of erosion of previously ovoid or spherical stones. Facetting indicates the existence of more than one stone. If only one facetted stone is found in an unopened specimen, others may have been passed into the common bile duct, and it is important that the surgeon is informed of the discovery.

After fixation, the specimen is measured if this has not been done already, and the mucosa, cut surface of the wall and serosa are examined. The mucosa of an inflamed gall bladder may have a variety of appearances. It will be pink and glistening if inflammation is slight or if a mucocele has formed. It may be red and granular because of hyperaemia in acute inflammation, white and firm when ulceration has healed by dense fibrosis, speckled yellow on a red or green background because of cholesterol accumulation in lamina propria macrophages (**42**), or black or green from deposition of bile pigments on or within the mucosa. There is usually fibrous thickening of the wall from chronic cholecystitis and this may be extensive in the fundus, mimicking neoplasia.

Carcinoma of the gall bladder is rare, and tends to occur at the fundus. It may form a solid white mass infiltrating the wall, or grow into the lumen as a soft, white, fronded tumour. There is usually a lymph node alongside the cystic duct, and there may be metastatic spread to this before the primary tumour is apparent macroscopically. It is therefore good practice to take a block of the node, when present, from all cholecystectomy specimens.

Where no focal disease is apparent, two blocks of the gall bladder, from the fundus and the neck, are usually sufficient to show the pathology present. Fragments of liver parenchyma attached to the serosa of the gall bladder should also be blocked, but local inflammatory changes often obscure any primary hepatic pathology which may be present.

Gall bladder: Macroscopical report

Type of specimen	Opened (or unopened) gall bladder, cystic duct, attached liver parenchyma
Measurements	Length and diameter at widest part
Description	
Serosa	Colour; presence of fat necrosis (which might indicate pancreatitis associated with stones in the common bile duct); presence and appearance of liver tissue on the serosa, cystic duct lymph node
Cut surface of wall	Thickness; colour; contour (distorted, constricted); consistency (firm, fibrosed, friable)
Mucosa	Colour; texture (granular, ulcerated, papillary); consistency (soft, friable)
Contents	Bile, mucus; number of stones and range of sizes (if there are very large numbers of tiny pigment stones, say this instead of counting them)

Example 42

The specimen consists of an opened gall bladder measuring 7 cm in length and 3.5 cm in maximum diameter. The serosa shows no significant abnormality. The wall thickness is uniform at 3 mm, and there are no focal lesions present. The mucosa has numerous tiny yellow patches on a background of velvety green tissue. The lumen contains thick green bile, and there are no stones. A single small lymph node is present adjacent to the cystic duct.

Blocks

- **A** fundus × 1
- **B** neck of gall bladder × 1
- **C** cystic duct lymph node × 1

40 An unopened cholecystectomy specimen. The serosal surface is congested and the thickness of the wall of the neck of the gall bladder is increased.

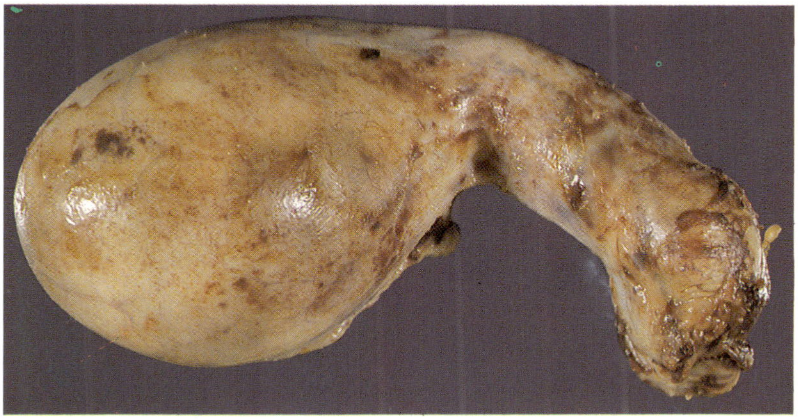

40

41 Specimen 40 opened longitudinally through the cystic duct. The mucosa is pale with irregular haemorrhagic areas. The lumen of the gall bladder contains facetted stones.

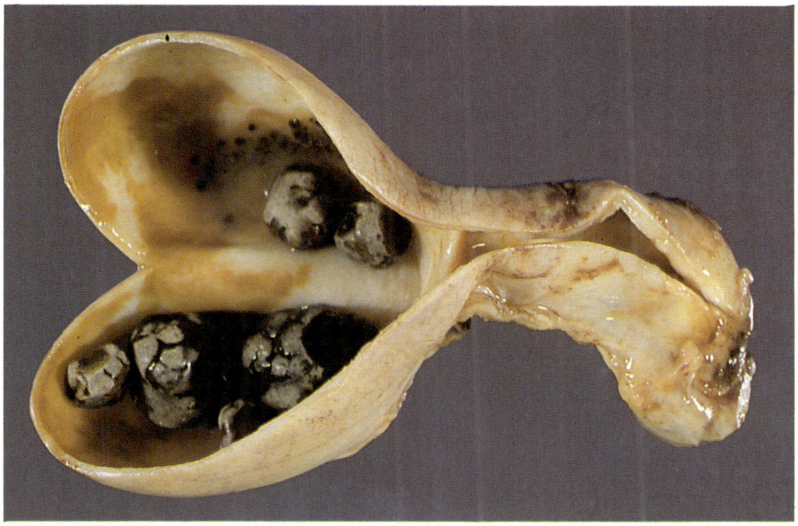

41

42 An opened gall bladder showing cholesterosis. The tiny yellow dots on the mucosa are due to collections of lipid-laden macrophages just below the epithelium.

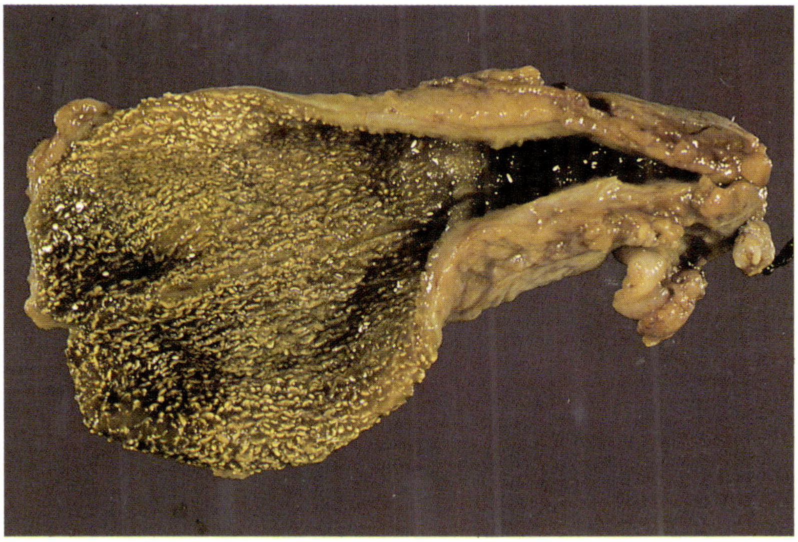

42

Exocrine pancreas

Small specimens

Needle biopsies of the pancreas may be performed when carcinoma of the pancreas is suspected. The biopsy is usually taken under direct vision at operation, but ultra-sound-directed biopsies are becoming more common. The specimen should be measured and described briefly ('A needle core of pale tissue measuring . . .'). The biopsy is embedded whole, and numerous levels should be requested.

Large specimens

Pancreatectomy is performed for malignant disease of the pancreas, and occasionally for severe chronic fibrosing pancreatitis. Distal pancreatectomy involves removal of the body and/or tail of the pancreas. This is usually for the treatment of endocrine tumours (p 117) and rarely for exocrine carcinomas of the pancreas.

The surgical treatment of lesions of the head of the pancreas is by Whipple's procedure. This involves excision of the distal part of the stomach and the duodenum, the proximal pancreas and the common bile duct as one block (**43a**).

Initial dissection

Distal pancreatectomy specimens are dealt with in Chapter 10.

Specimens from a Whipple's operation can appear complicated because of the number of organs involved, but are usually easy to orientate, especially if received unfixed. If possible, the specimen should be examined in the presence of the surgeons who performed the operation. The excision margins of the pancreas and common bile duct, and the external surface of the specimen in the region of the tumour, should be identified and marked with India ink. The hollow viscera are opened along the greater curve of stomach, across the anterior wall of the pylorus and down the lateral aspect of the duodenum (**44**). The tissues can then be pinned out onto a cork board so that the anatomical relations of the organs are preserved. The specimen should be photographed if possible.

Dissection of specimen

Dissection of a Whipple's operation specimen depends on the site of the tumour. Most commonly it will be in the periampullary region, but occasionally it may be more peripheral, for example, in the superior part of the head of the pancreas and involving the greater curve of the stomach.

Before the specimen is dissected further, it is important to identify, remove and carefully label the sites of lymph nodes taken for microscopical examination. A search should be made for lymph nodes on the serosa of the duodenum, the greater and lesser curves of the stomach, over the surface of the pancreas and around the common bile duct.

In most cases it is possible to detach the stomach from the main specimen by cutting across the pylorus, antrum or body where the stomach is clearly uninvolved by tumour. Similarly, the duodenum distal to the site of involvement of the tumour may be detached and examined separately.

The remaining specimen will consist of the pancreas, the duodenum adjacent to the pancreas and the biliary system. It is useful to take blocks from the excision margins at this stage, before the specimen is distorted by further dissection. Blocks should be taken from the resection margins of the pancreas (**45, 46**) and the common bile duct, and from the exterior surface of the specimen if this appears to be involved or approached by tumour. The common bile duct is then opened longitudinally, as far as possible into the area of the tumour, with fine scissors.

When the distal 1 cm of the pancreas has been removed for blocking the excision margin, in most cases the pancreatic duct will be visible on the cut surface. A fine probe can be inserted into the duct and gently advanced as far as possible towards the duodenum to see if the duct is patent. The head of the pancreas should then be incised with a long-bladed knife coronally at right angles to the duodenal mucosa. If the probe has passed through the ampulla of Vater into the lumen of the duodenum it can be used to guide the knife blade. This manoeuvre usually displays the relations of a tumour with the duodenum and pancreas. Alternatively, if the duct is obliterated by tumour, sagittal slices parallel to the excision line can be made into the head of the pancreas (**46**). Blocks are then taken to show the tumour and its relations with the duodenum, common bile duct, the rest of the pancreas, and surrounding adipose tissues (**43b**).

It is important to try to determine the site of origin of a carcinoma, as the prognosis of periampullary carcinoma is better than for carcinoma elsewhere in the head of the pancreas. However, in practice it may not be possible to determine whether the tumour has arisen from the common bile duct, the terminal pancreatic duct or the duodenal papilla.

Exocrine pancreas: Macroscopical report

Type of specimen	Partial pancreatectomy, distal pancreatectomy, Whipple's operation specimen (comprising . . .)
Measurements	
Organs	Stomach (lengths of greater and lesser curvatures); spleen (weight and dimensions); length of duodenum; length and maximum thickness of pancreas; length of common bile duct
Description	
Tumour	Number (single or multifocal); site (head, body, tail; in duodenum, common bile duct, gastric wall, spleen); size (maximum diameter of tumour, size of exophytic portion within duodenum, if present) or range of sizes if multifocal; colour; contour (exophytic, papillary, infiltrative, circumscribed, multifocal); consistency (hard, gritty, cystic, soft); distance of the tumour from excision margins
Rest of specimen	Pancreas away from tumour (fibrosed, calcified, haemorrhagic, dilatation of ducts); biliary system away from tumour (dilatation, fibrosis, congestion, presence of calculi); stomach, duodenum, spleen, omentum and other tissues present

Example 43-46

A Whipple's operation specimen consisting of the gastric antrum, the duodenum, the distal common bile duct and part of the head of the pancreas. The stomach is 7.2 cm along the lesser curve and 11.1 cm along the greater curve. The duodenum is 20 cm long. The common bile duct is 2.5 cm long, and has a maximum diameter of 1.7 cm. The head of the pancreas measures 2.5 × 2.5 × 5 cm.

There is a nodular mass 1.2 cm in diameter indenting the duodenum at the level of the duodenal papilla. There is no overlying ulceration, and no other mucosal abnormality is apparent. Sections through the ampulla of Vater show an ill-defined tumour mass involving the distal 2 cm of the common bile duct and adjacent pancreatic tissue. The entire tumour measures 2.7 × 1.5 × 2.5 cm. Its cut surface is white with several cystic foci containing translucent mucoid material. The tumour appears macroscopically to extend to the pancreatic resection margin, but has not spread to the excision line of the common bile duct or into the peripancreatic adipose tissue.

There is no apparent abnormality in the stomach, and the duodenum away from the area of the ampulla appears normal. Seven greater curve lymph nodes, four lesser curve nodes, five peripancreatic nodes and two nodes from the lower end of the common bile duct are identified. ►

Blocks

A pancreatic excision margins × 2
B common bile duct resection margin × 1
C tumour × 2
D tumour and ampulla of Vater × 1
E tumour and common bile duct × 1
F tumour, surface of pancreas and adjacent adipose tissue × 3
G gastric excision margin × 1
H gastric antrum × 1
J first part of duodenum × 1
K third part of duodenum × 1
L distal excision margin × 1
M lymph nodes from greater curve × 7
N lymph nodes from lesser curve × 4
P lymph nodes from surface of pancreas × 5
R lymph nodes from lower end of common bile duct × 2

43a

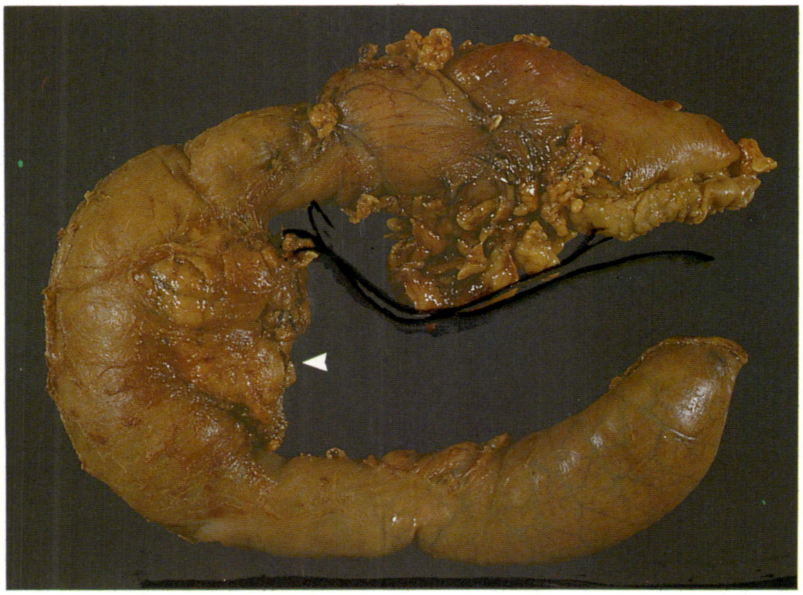

43a An intact specimen removed at a Whipple's operation. This consists of the gastric antrum, the duodenum and proximal jejunum, and the head of the pancreas (▶). The tumour is difficult to see but easy to locate by palpation in the pancreas and adjacent duodenal wall.

43b

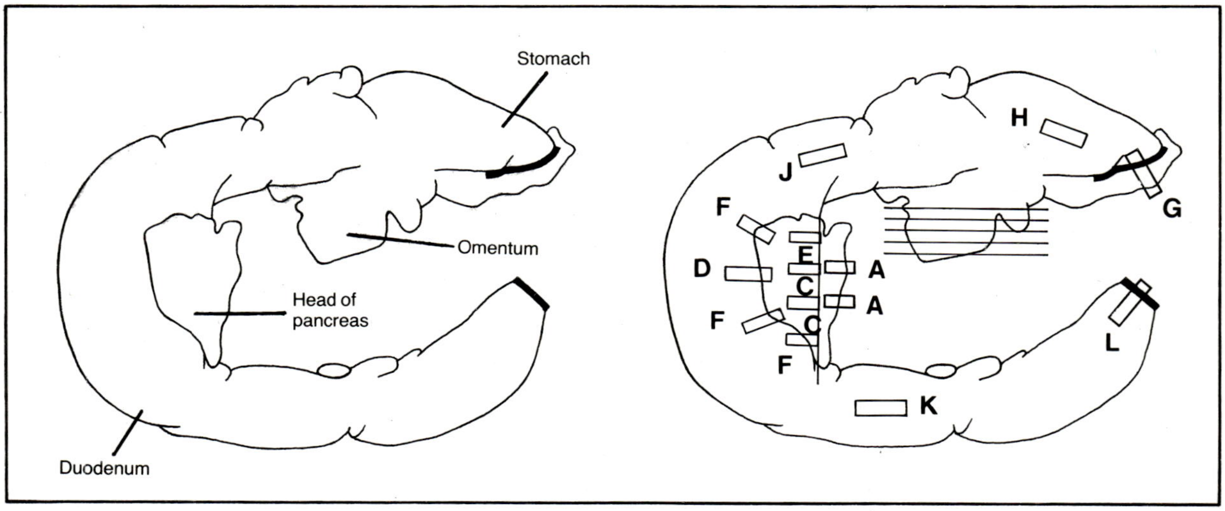

43b Blocks taken from a Whipple's operation specimen: pancreatic excision margin (**A**); common bile duct excision margin (**B**—not shown); centre of tumour (**C**); tumour and ampulla of Vater (**D**); tumour and common bile duct (**E**); tumour and surface of pancreas and adjacent adipose tissue (**F**); gastric excision margin (**G**); gastric antrum (**H**); first part of duodenum (**J**); third part of duodenum (**K**); distal excision margin (**L**); lymph nodes from greater curve (**M**); lymph nodes from lesser curve (**N**—not shown); lymph nodes from surface of pancreas (**P**—not shown); lymph nodes from lower end of common bile duct (**R**—not shown).

44 Specimen 43, with the stomach and duodenum opened to show the indentation of the area of the duodenal papilla by the tumour in the head of pancreas (▶).

44

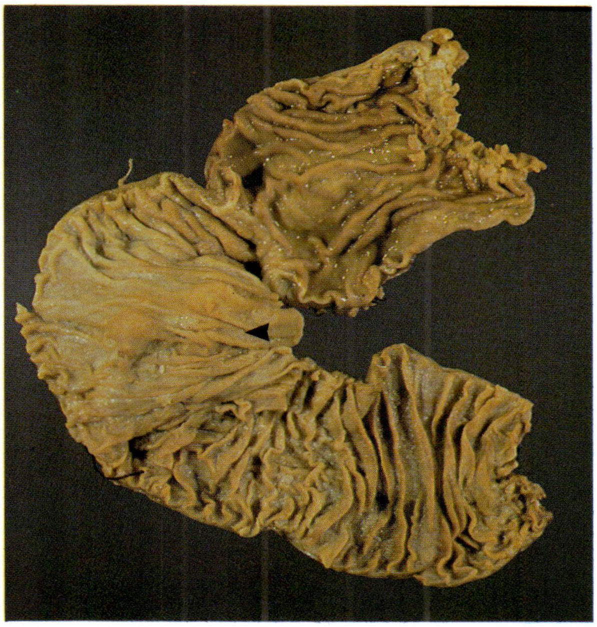

45 Specimen 43 from the serosal aspect. The pancreatic tumour can be seen after the removal of the distal excision margin of the pancreas.

45

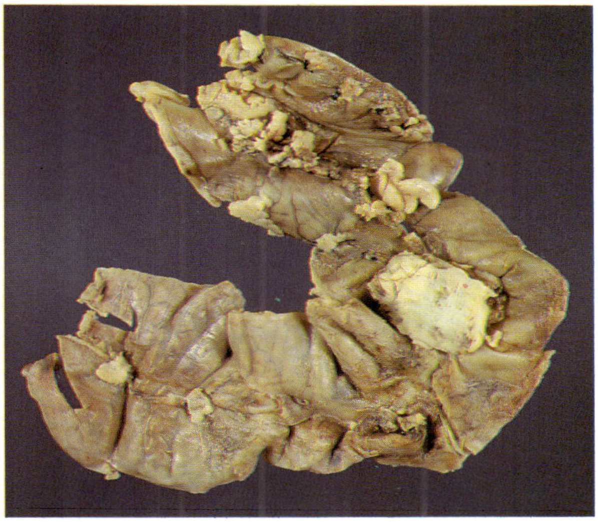

46 A sagittal slice through the tumour in 45, the medial aspect at the pancreatic resection end. The tumour has occluded the common bile duct (▶) and completely obliterated the pancreatic duct.

46

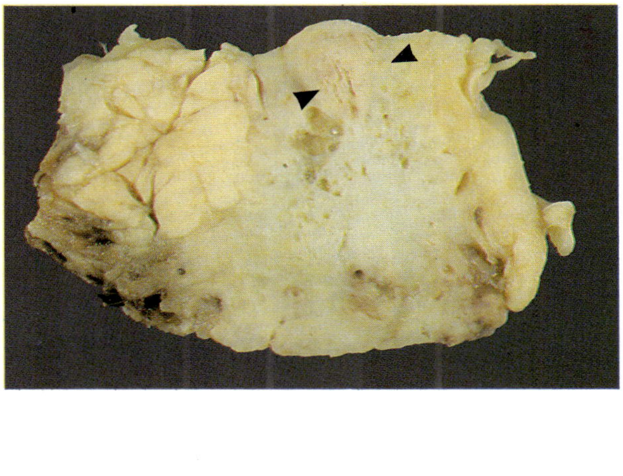

CHAPTER 3
FEMALE GENITAL SYSTEM

Vulva

Small specimens

Small specimens taken from the skin and mucosa of the vulva should be treated in the same way as skin biopsies from elsewhere in the body (p 97).

Large specimens

Types of specimen
Vulvectomy is performed for malignancy and for the symptomatic relief of lichen sclerosus and other inflammatory conditions. The operation ranges from excision of one labium majus and adjacent skin to removal of the entire vulva (**47**). Inguinal extensions to include lymph nodes and perineal extensions around the anus may also be included (**48-50**).

Initial dissection
Specimens are often received unfixed or only partly fixed. They should be measured, then if necessary pinned out onto a cork board for further fixation.

Dissection of specimen
After fixation the specimen should be photographed. Measurements should be taken if they have not been made before fixation. The inguinal wings of the specimen are best examined first. Starting laterally and progressing medially along the deep aspect of the specimen, the adipose tissue is palpated, then close cuts are made through the fat to look for lymph nodes (p 15). Half of any node found in the specimen should be blocked, keeping those from the right and left separate. If the skin is left intact, the slices will remain in sequence.

After the lymph nodes have been harvested, the vulva is dissected. Parallel cuts should be made through any focal lesion and immediately adjacent skin or mucosa to demonstrate its deep and lateral extensions. Blocks should be taken from the lesion, underlying tissues, and deep and lateral excision margins. If a large condylomatous (warty) lesion is present, numerous blocks

Vulva: Macroscopical report	
Type of specimen	Labium majus or minus, hemivulvectomy, total vulvectomy, extended vulvectomy with inguinal and perineal extension
Measurements	Width of the specimen Distance from the pubic (superior) aspect to the posterior perineal limit Length of vagina from the base of the labia minora to the deep excision line
Description	
Lesions	Focal, diffuse (widespread, extensive) Size; site; distance from excision margins and from clitoris Colour; consistency (firm, hard, boggy, friable, indurated, oedematous); texture of surface (roughened, ulcerated, crusted, atrophic, granular), appearance of borders of lesion
Other tissues	Appearance of vulva, inguinal skin, perineum, etc. away from lesion Appearance of the underlying tissues Lymph nodes

from the deep borders should be taken; diagnosis of a verrucous carcinoma can be very difficult even with extensive sampling. Incisions to examine the suprapubic or superior margins, the vaginal and perineal margins and the lateral inguinal margins should be made along the lines of shortest distance from the lesion to the excision line. More than one block may be necessary. Skin from the vulva contralateral to the lesion should be blocked, and the clitoris and clitoral area in line with the nearest extension of the lesion should also be carefully sampled (**48b, 50b**).

Example 48-50

The specimen is a radical vulvectomy consisting of vulva, vagina, inguinal skin and underlying tissues. It measures 28 cm in maximum width and 9.1 cm from the suprapubic resection margin to the perineal aspect. The central vulval area measures 10 × 9 cm and there is underlying tissue to a depth of 3 cm. The inguinal nodes and surrounding adipose tissue measure approximately 8 × 6 × 2 cm on each side. The distance from the base of the labia minora to the vaginal excision line is 1.4 cm.

On the upper aspect of the right labium majus is a nodular white tumour mass 2.5 cm in diameter. On cut sections this appears to extend close to but not up to the deep excision line immediately below the tumour, and to spread to 1.7 cm away from the base of the clitoris. The vaginal, suprapubic, lateral, and perineal excision lines are well clear of the tumour. The skin of the left labium and of the right labium below the tumour has a shiny white surface. The skin elsewhere shows no significant abnormality.

Twelve lymph nodes are present in the left inguinal wing of the specimen, ranging in size from 1.2-3 cm in diameter. Eight lymph nodes are found in the right inguinal wing, and have a similar range of sizes.

Blocks

- **A** suprapubic resection line × 1
- **B** right lateral resection line × 1
- **C** left lateral resection line × 1
- **D** perineal resection line × 1
- **E** right inguinal nodes × 8
- **F** left inguinal nodes × 12
- **G** tumour and deep resection line × 2
- **H** tumour and vaginal resection line × 2
- **J** clitoris × 1
- **K** contralateral vulva × 1

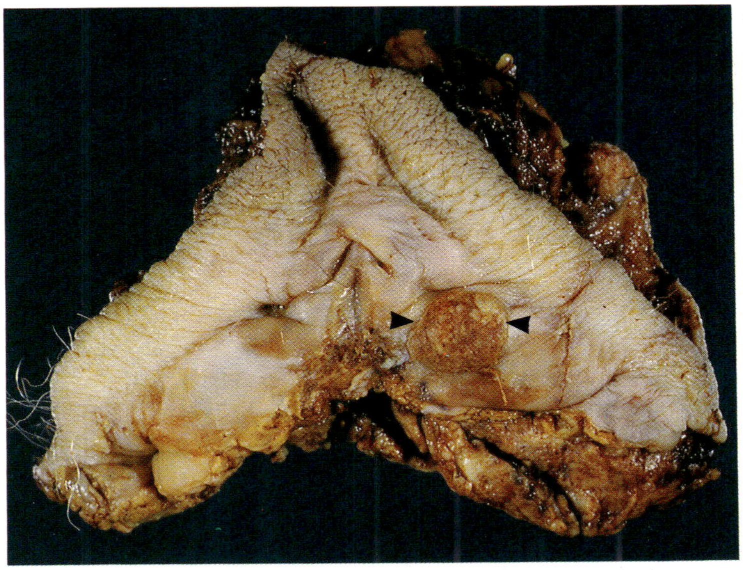

47 A simple vulvectomy specimen with an ulcerated carcinoma on the left labium minus (▶). The surrounding skin and the skin of the right labium minus are smooth and shiny. The latter was found to be due to lichen sclerosus.

47

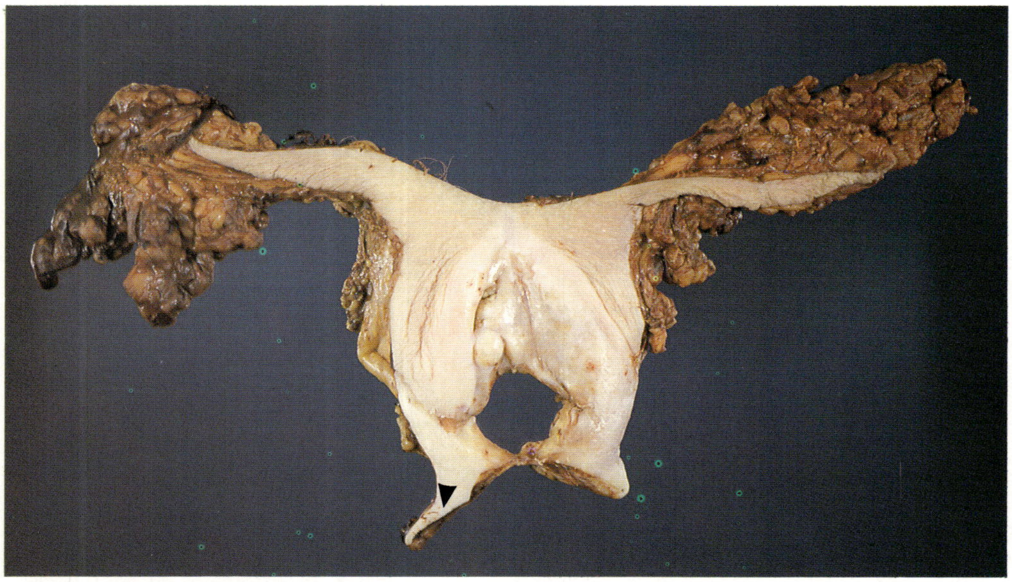

48a A radical vulvectomy specimen with inguinal skin, radical node dissection and right perineal extension (▶).

48b

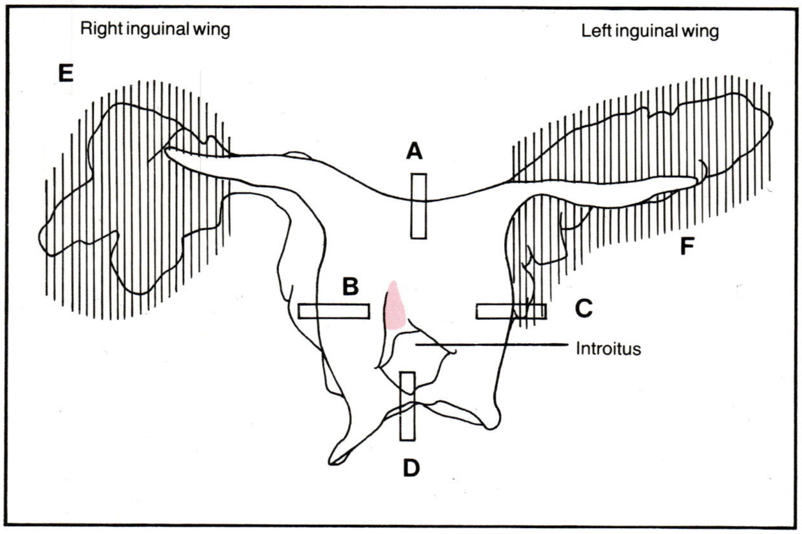

48b Blocks taken from a vulvectomy specimen, Part 1 (for Part 2, see 50b): suprapubic excision margin (**A**); right lateral excision margin (**B**); left lateral excision margin (**C**); perineal excision margin (**D**); right inguinal lymph nodes (**E**); left inguinal lymph nodes (**F**).

49

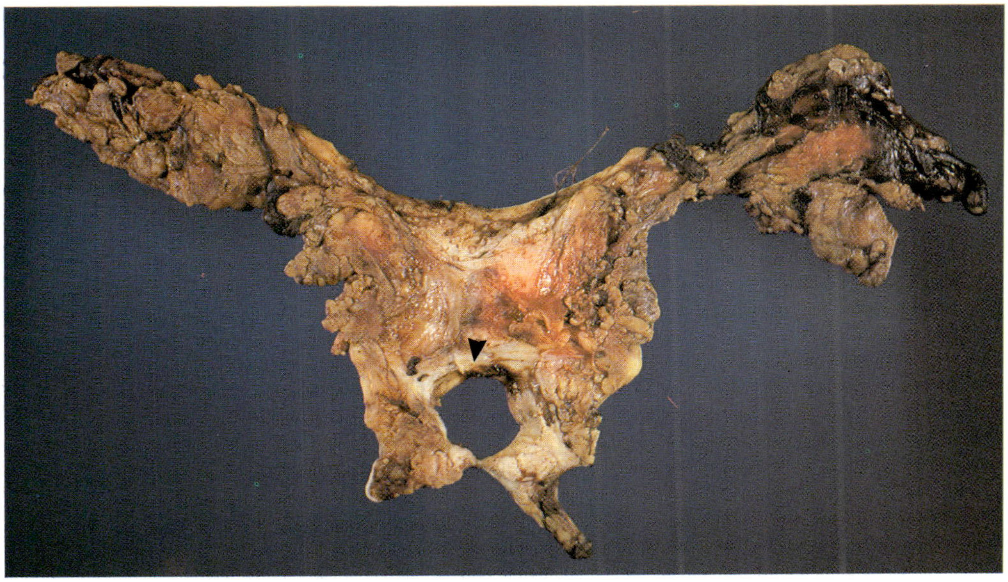

49 The reverse of 48 showing the vaginal excision margin (▶).

50a

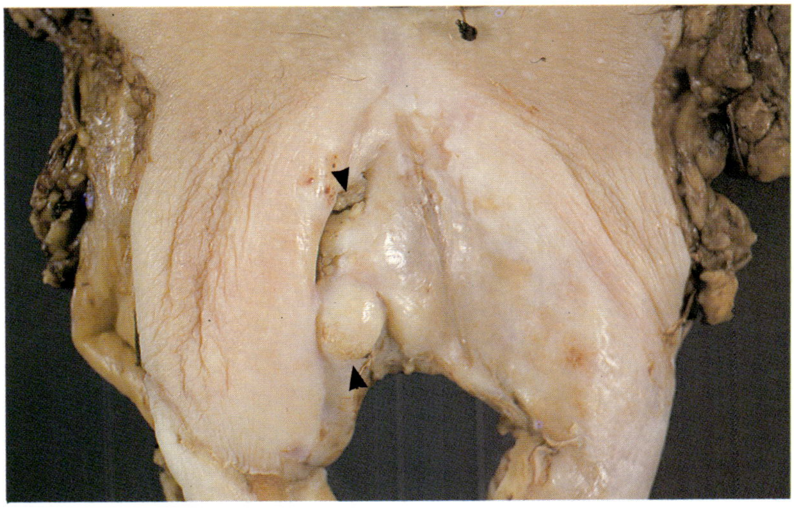

50a A detail of 48. There is a white, nodular tumour mass in the superior part of the right labium minus (▶), extending from just below the clitoris to the edge of the introitus. The skin of the left labium shows areas of irregular white thickening.

50b

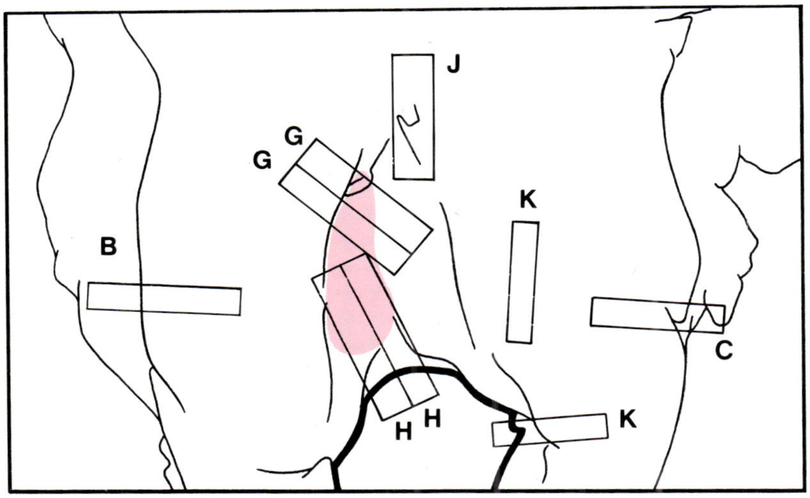

50b Blocks taken from a vulvectomy specimen, Part 2: tumour plus deep excision margin (**G**); tumour and vaginal excision margin (**H**); clitoris (**J**); contralateral vulva (**K**). (**B** and **C** correspond to **48b**.)

Cervix

Small specimens

Curettings

Irregular fragments may be removed from the endocervical canal for a variety of reasons, including the investigation of inflammatory and neoplastic conditions. Polypoid masses should be embedded whole if possible (**51**). If they are composed largely of mucus this should be recorded, as it will explain why the histological sections show very little epithelium or stroma. Curettings may be taken specifically of the endocervix or may be obtained during endometrial curettage. These cervical specimens are treated as for endometrial curettings (see below).

Biopsies

Colposcopically directed biopsies of the ectocervix and endocervix are taken for similar reasons as curettings. They vary in size and can be difficult to orientate. As with other specimens from body surfaces, precise embedding is essential so that sections can be cut at right angles to the epithelium.

If the biopsy is relatively large (more than 5 mm) it can be bisected at right angles to the epithelial surface. The margins of excision are seldom critical as the procedure is usually simply a diagnostic test, but it is important that all of the tissue is blocked and numerous sections are examined. Specimens from different areas should be embedded separately.

Cone and cylinder biopsy of the cervix

Cone biopsy, where the tissue is excised with a scalpel, is the most common method of sampling the ectocervix, squamocolumnar junction and endocervical canal together (**52a**). This type of biopsy is taken for investigation and sometimes for treatment of intraepithelial neoplasia or microinvasive carcinoma. When laser light is used to excise tissue, it produces a domed cylinder rather than a cone, and the lateral borders are covered by charred debris. The dissection of both is similar.

Dissection

There are several different methods of handling a cone biopsy specimen, and many variations on each method. All provide similar information. The common aim is to demonstrate the presence and extent of dysplasia/neoplasia and to assess whether excision is complete.

Cone biopsies are usually received unfixed, and may have a suture marker placed in the most anterior aspect ('12 o'clock' position) (**52a, 53a**). The excision margins can be painted with India ink so that they are easily recognizable on the sections. The commonest way to block a cone biopsy is to open it through the endocervical canal; the cut can be made at the site of the suture marker or, if the external os is slit-shaped, at one pole of the slit. The latter will display a wide expanse of the squamocolumnar junction (it is unwise to assume that the long axis of the os always divides the anterior and posterior aspects - a slit-shaped os may run anteroposteriorly). If the cone is irregular or eccentric, it should be opened through the thinnest or shortest part. The specimen is then pinned out onto a cork board to fix (**53a**). Suture markers should be left in place so that the '12 o'clock' position can be identified when blocks are taken.

All of the tissue excised in a cone biopsy is submitted for histological examination.

Small biopsies: Macroscopical report	
Site	'One o'clock', 'six o'clock' (**56**) endocervical biopsy, polyp, posterior fornix, etc.
Measurements	Number of fragments from each site Size or range of sizes Greatest dimension if very small
Description	Colour Contour (irregular, round, a strip of . . .) Consistency (mucoid, firm, papillary)

Cone biopsy: Macroscopical report

Type of specimen	Short cone, long cone, domed cylinder
Measurements	Diameter and/or circumference of the ectocervical face Size and shape of external os Length of endocervical canal from squamocolumnar junction to tip of cone
Description	
Ectocervix	Colour; texture (smooth, granular); contour; focal lesions
Squamocolumnar junction	Position and appearance of squamocolumnar junction (at external os, over ectocervical face, within canal, indistinct, marked by iodine, ulcerated)
Endocervix	Colour; texture (papillary, ulcerated); focal lesions

Example 52-53
The specimen consists of a long cone biopsy of the cervix measuring 2.7 cm across its ectocervical face and 2 cm from the external os to the endocervical excision margin. The os is slit-shaped and is 1.3 cm long. The endocervical canal shows no apparent macroscopical abnormality. The ectocervix shows an irregular granular area of red mucosa extending 0.5 cm around the external os, compatible with eversion.

Blocks
15 blocks (A-R) taken clockwise from the suture marker around the entire specimen. All embedded.

Blocks from a cone biopsy should be about 2-3 mm thick; if they are less, they have a tendency to curl and will not provide good sections. The wedge-shaped blocks (**53b**, **54**) are labelled sequentially, and the block from the area of the suture marker should be given the first number or letter in the sequence. On large cones it may be possible to obtain 15-20 blocks (**55**). Each block is placed in the processing cassette so that the correct face is sectioned (**53b-55**). On the final report, the sites of lesions in the cone are indicated by reference to the time-honoured clock face (**56**).

A problem with this method arises when the cone biopsy is received fixed, as it is harder to take blocks which include both endocervical and ectocervical mucosa. In this case, another method is to leave the cone biopsy intact and take parallel sagittal sections about 3 mm apart through the entire specimen. Blocks are labelled sequentially, and numerous sections are taken from those which pass through the endocervical canal (**52b**). This method allows easier reconstruction of the three-dimensional appearances of the ectocervix and can be related to colposcopic findings. Though useful in research departments, and when the cone is inadvertently fixed whole, it has, however, found little favour in routine practice.

51

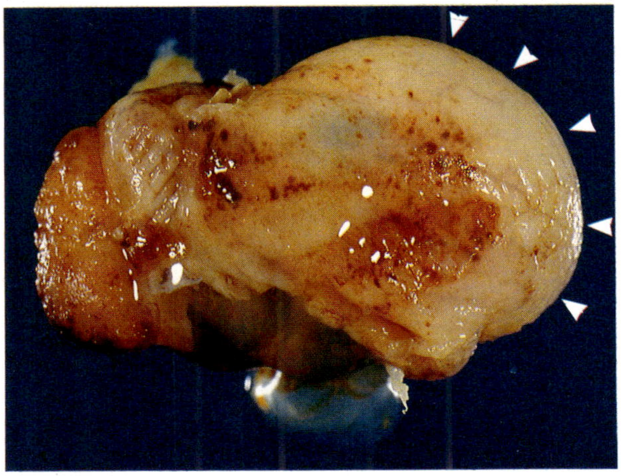

51 An endocervical polyp, covered in part by clear mucus. Much of the surface is smooth and white because of squamous metaplasia (▶).

52a

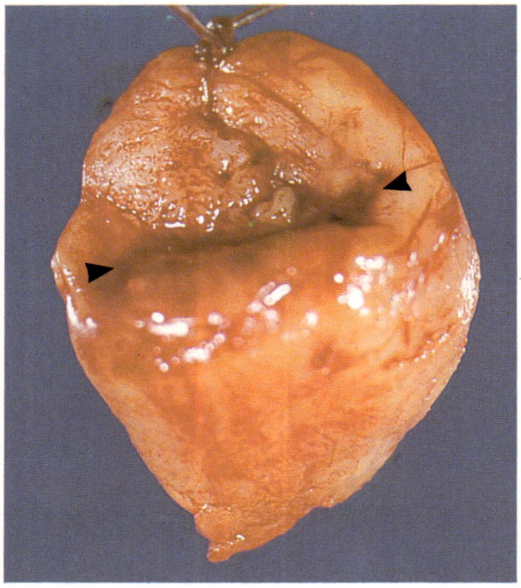

52b

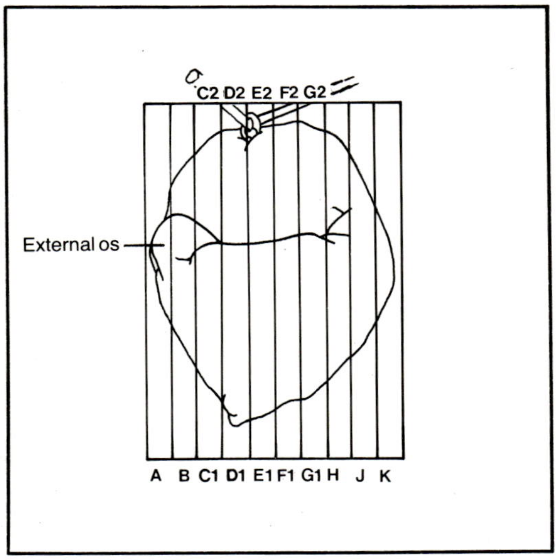

52a A cone biopsy of the cervix. The '12 o'clock' position (i.e. the most anterior aspect of the biopsy) has been marked by the gynaecologist with a suture. In this case, the external cervical os is slit-shaped and easily identified (▶).

52b Blocks taken from a cone biopsy. When it is not possible to open a cone biopsy and fix it properly, or when the canal cannot be identified, parallel sagittal cuts are made and the blocks are laid out as shown. If blocks become halved because cuts pass through the endocervical canal, the tissue should be labelled appropriately, e.g. C1 and C2.

53a

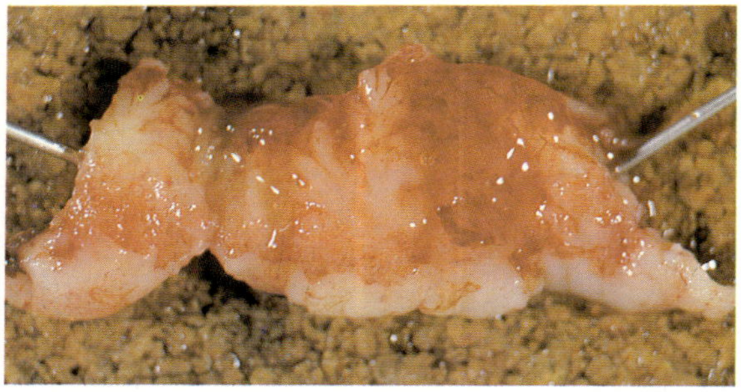

53a The cone biopsy 52a opened, with the suture marker still in place. The tissue is attached to a cork board, pinned through the cervical stroma rather than the epithelial surface.

53b

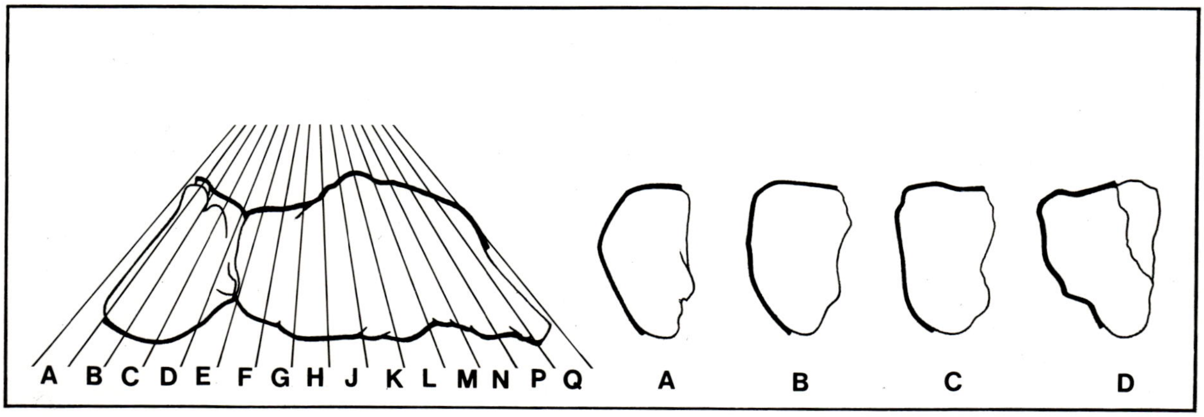

53b Sequential cuts through the opened cone biopsy. Each block should be as complete a cross section of the cone as possible, and should be neither too thin nor too thick. It is better to aim for well-shaped blocks than for large numbers of them.

54 and 55 Sequential slices of tissue. As each slice of tissue is removed it is laid on the cutting board or placed directly into cassettes in the correct orientation, so that when sections are cut sampling will be at regular intervals.

54

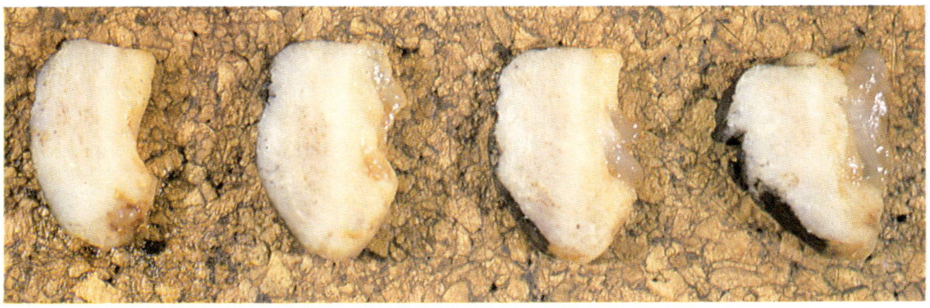

55

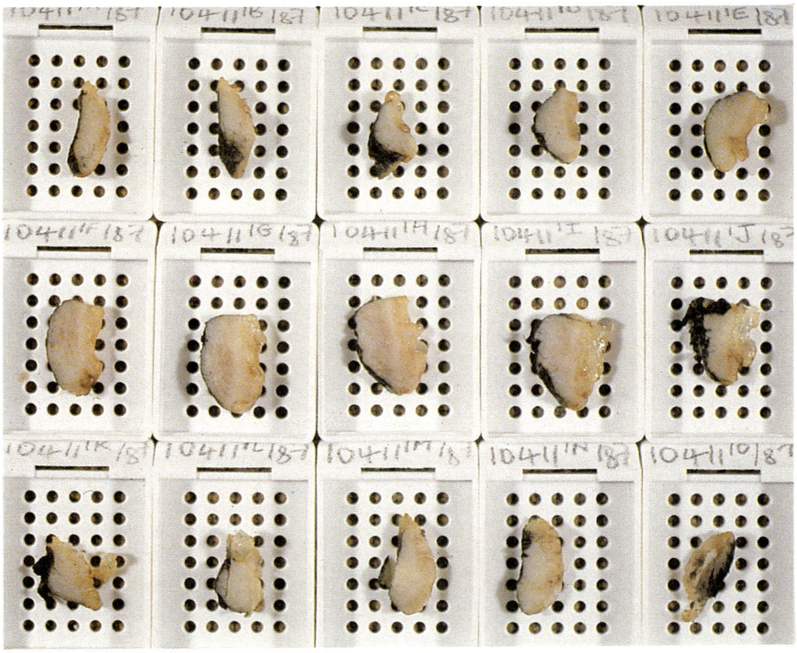

56 Clock faces. The inner ring of letters corresponds to the sequentially lettered blocks from a cone biopsy, and will vary in number depending on the number of blocks taken. The regions in which disease is found histologically can be reported in relation to the clock face. For example, if 15 blocks (labelled A-R) are taken and CIN3 is found on sections between E and N, the report might read 'CIN3 is present on tissue between the four and eleven o'clock positions'.

56

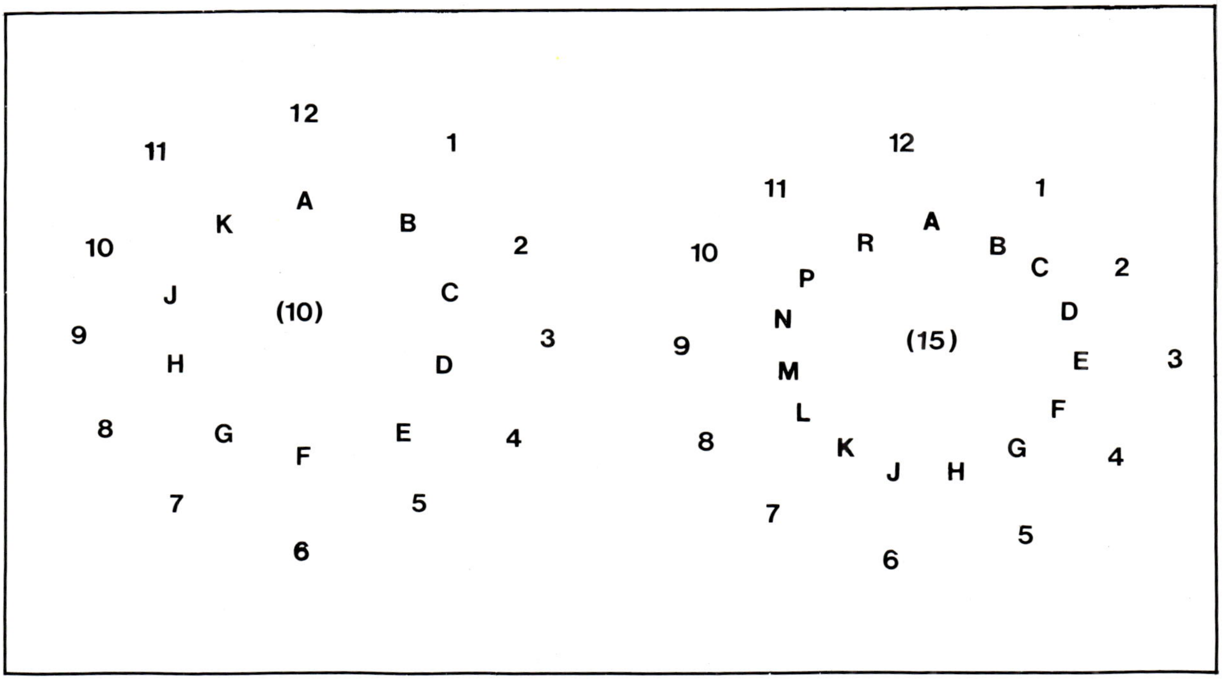

Uterine corpus

Small specimens

About one third of all histopathology specimens received in a general histopathology laboratory are gynaecological, and a large proportion of these are from the endometrium. Uterine curettage is performed for a variety of reasons, but the commonest is bleeding *per vaginam*. The endometrial causes include hormonal imbalance, inflammation, hyperplasia and neoplasia.

The entire specimen of endometrial curettings is embedded unless the amount is very large. An assessment should be made of the amount received, either by measurement of the aggregated specimen in millimetres or by eye, recording the quantity as scanty, moderate or copious. It is worthwhile remarking on the presence of obviously polypoid fragments at this stage. They may be less easily recognizable on histological sections, and should be embedded separately.

Tissue from spontaneous and therapeutic abortions and from evacuation of retained products of conception varies in amount from small fragments to large quantities of tissue with recognizable fetal parts. Chorionic villi may be readily visible as white papillary fragments which sometimes surround a recognizable gestation sac (**57**); if not, these should be sought in pale solid areas enclosed in blood clot. It is important to establish that normal villi are present and, where macroscopical identification of villi is difficult, it is better to take several blocks on the first occasion than to have to return to the specimen later. Villi from a hydatidiform mole are swollen, rounded vesicles ranging in size from a few millimetres to over a centimetre (**58, 59**).

Pale pink, spongy decidua is usually present as irregular tissue fragments. Sometimes a decidual cast is received, a cystic ovoid body about 3 cm long formed from the entire decidual lining of the pregnant uterus.
Fibroids (leiomyomas) may be removed by myomectomy to preserve the uterus. They should be measured, sectioned and described. A portion of each should be submitted for histology (**60, 61**).

Large specimens

Hysterectomy may be performed for dysfunctional uterine bleeding, certain inflammatory conditions, and cervical, endometrial, myometrial, tubal and ovarian neoplasia. Depending on the indication for hysterectomy, the uterus may be excised alone or with attached vagina, fallopian tubes, ovaries, parametria and occasionally

Endometrium: Macroscopical report	
Site and type of specimen	Endometrial curettings, products of conception, endocervical curettings
Measurements	Curettings (scanty, moderate, copious), or dimensions of aggregated tissue
Description	Polypoid fragments, irregular brown fragments Papillary fragments of chorionic villi, fetal parts, blood clot, sheets of spongy pink tissue, thin-walled vesicles containing clear fluid

Fibroids: Macroscopical report	
Measurements	Number and diameter of fibroids
Description	Colour (pale pink, white, red) Consistency (rubbery, calcified, soft) Cut surface (whorled, homogeneous, focally necrotic)

other tissues. A simple hysterectomy specimen will consist of the uterus and cervix, with or without a short cuff of vagina (**62**). An extended hysterectomy will involve removal of the fallopian tubes, ovaries and parametrium as well (**63**). A Wertheim's extended hysterectomy with pelvic lymphadenectomy involves the removal of the iliac, obturator and para-aortic lymph nodes, which should be sent to the laboratory in separately labelled containers.

Initial dissection

It is essential that the clinical details of a case are known before the specimen is dissected. The procedure used will depend on whether the specimen is received fresh or fixed, intact or opened, and on the suspected or proven pathology — for example, dissection for fibroids will be quite different from dissection for cervical neoplasia.

Hysterectomy specimens may be orientated in several ways:

- the gynaecologist may have opened the uterus longitudinally through the anterior surface to help fixation (**62**)
- the insertion of the fallopian tubes is towards the posterior aspect of the fundus, and the round ligament lies anteriorly (**63**)
- the peritoneum covers only the corpus anteriorly but overlaps the cervix posteriorly (**63, 64**).

If a hysterectomy has been performed for cervical neoplasia, first the vagina and then the cervix should be detached. The cervix should be opened and treated as for a cone biopsy (see above). The corpus is then opened as described below.

When the uterus is received intact, it may be opened by cutting through the endocervical canal and endometrial cavity along one lateral border to the point of entry of the fallopian tube. A probe inserted through the cervix into the cavity may be useful as a guide. The endocervical canal and the endometrial cavity are then inspected, and where suitable the cut is continued down the contralateral border to bisect the specimen. This technique does not distort the flat anterior and posterior walls of the cavity (**65, 67a** and **b**).

Another way of opening the uterus is to make a cut through the anterior wall of the cervix and uterus (**62**). A wick of cotton wool may be inserted in the uterine cavity or the specimen may need to be propped open with a small length of perspex rod to help fixation.

Dissection of specimen

After fixation and photography, the uterus should be described and measured. In most departments the specimen (without the adnexa) is also weighed, but the range of normal uterine weight is wide and the significance of this measurement is therefore doubtful.

The cervix and vaginal cuff are removed, if still attached at this stage, by a cut through the isthmus. For non-neoplastic disease two blocks of the cervix are usually sufficient, preferably from the anterior and posterior aspects.

Close transverse cuts should then be made through the corpus. If a strip of serosa is left uncut the sections will remain in sequence. Sagittal incisions may be made instead of transverse ones, but those from the lateral aspects will have no endometrium on them and orientation may therefore prove more difficult.

Hysterectomy for carcinoma

In a case of total hysterectomy for invasive cervical, endometrial, tubal and ovarian carcinoma, bilateral salpingo-oophorectomy and omentectomy will usually be performed; in a Wertheim's procedure for cervical carcinoma, the regional lymph nodes are also dissected. It is important to establish the upper, lower and deep limits of the tumour and its relation to the resection margins. In patients who have been treated with radiotherapy pre-operatively, the resulting fibrosis may make it impossible to determine the extent of the tumour spread by naked eye examination, and this may only become apparent on microscopy. Carefully labelled blocks are essential in these cases if orientation is to be preserved.

In some hospitals, the management of

endometrial carcinoma is dictated by the depth of penetration of the tumour through the myometrium. It is therefore important to establish the maximum depth of extension of the tumour into the myometrium. Several blocks should be taken of the full thickness of the wall. If they are too large to embed whole they should be bisected, and the two halves correspondingly labelled (**67c**). It can be very difficult to determine the proportion of the thickness of myometrium occupied by the tumour when the inner layers of the muscle have been replaced by malignant cells. If the tumour is localized, the thickness of the myometrium before invasion can be estimated from a block taken from the corresponding uninvolved contralateral uterine wall. Once the local extent of the tumour has been established, the rest of the specimen, with any nodes sent separately, and the omentum, should be examined for metastases.

Hysterectomy for fibroids

There is wide variation in the number of blocks considered necessary from a fibroid uterus. Each fibroid (leiomyoma) over 5 mm in diameter should be examined microscopically, and with large fibroids more than one block will be necessary (**68a, 68b**). The number will depend on the macroscopical appearances — where necrosis, haemorrhage, lack of circumscription or other atypical features are found in a fibroid, more blocks will be necessary. Blocks should also be taken from the endometrium, cervix and adnexa, if present (**68b**).

Hysterectomy for non-neoplastic disease

In non-neoplastic disease, as well as the

Hysterectomy: Macroscopical report	
(either) **Type of specimen**	Simple hysterectomy, extended hysterectomy, Wertheim's hysterectomy with pelvic lymphadenectomy
(or) **List of tissues present**	Vagina, cervix, uterus, fallopian tubes, ovaries Omentum and lymph nodes (which may be sent separately)
(and) **Measurements**	Weight of specimen Length from ectocervix to top of fundus Length of vaginal cuff, if present Anteroposterior and transverse measurements of fundus at widest part
Description	
Focal lesions	*Type of lesion* Polyp, fibroid, ulcer, tumour *Site* Endometrial, submucosal, intramural, subserosal, extending into the endocervical canal *Number and size* Diameter if spherical, or maximum dimensions *Shape* Pedunculated, sessile *Colour and consistency* Soft, friable, rubbery *Cut surface* Whorled, variegated, haemorrhagic, cystic, calcified, circumscribed
Other tissues	
Vagina	Colour; texture
Ectocervix	Colour; texture (smooth, velvety, glistening); contour (nodular with Nabothian cysts, scarred and distorted)
Endocervix	Colour; texture
Endometrium	Thickness; colour
Myometrium	Thickness; colour; uniformity
Serosa	Colour; contour (distorted by leiomyomas, scarred, focal nodules of tumour or endometriosis, ruptured); texture (fibrinous exudate, granular) Appearance of parametrium, peritoneum lining the pouch of Douglas
Fallopian tubes, ovaries	*(see next sections, below)*

standard anterior and posterior blocks of the cervix, blocks should be taken if possible from the anterior or posterior walls of the uterus where the endometrium is relatively linear. A block should be taken of the endometrium, underlying myometrium and serosa. In small, atrophic uteri it may be possible to embed this as one block but in larger specimens it should be bisected.

Example 66-67

A uterus measuring 9.8 cm from fundus to 7.1 cm between the horns and 5.3 cm anteroposteriorly, together with attached tubes and ovaries. The uterus without the adnexa weighs 60 g.

The peritoneal covering is smooth and shiny. On opening the specimen there is a soft tumour mass within the uterine cavity, 3 × 2.1 × 2.2 cm in maximum dimensions, which has a papillary surface and is composed of soft white tissue. This extends into the outer third of the myometrium on the left, with a maximum thickness of 2.3 cm. At one point it is only 0.6 cm from the overlying serosa. The myometrium away from the tumour is 2.6 cm wide at its maximum. The ecto- and endocervix show no macroscopic abnormality.

The fallopian tubes are both 4 cm in length and 0.3 cm in maximum diameter. The right ovary measures 2.2 × 1.3 × 1 cm in maximum dimensions, and the left 2 × 1.3 × 1.2 cm. No evidence of tumour or other abnormality is noted in the adnexa.

Blocks

- **A** anterior cervix × 1
- **B** posterior cervix × 1
- **C1** endometrial aspect of tumour and uterine wall × 1
- **C2** serosal aspect of tumour and uterine wall × 1
- **D** tumour × 1
- **E** tumour and isthmus × 2
- **F** uninvolved endometrium, myometrium and serosa × 1
- **G** right ovary and fallopian tube with parametrium × 2
- **H** left ovary and fallopian tube with parametrium × 2

57

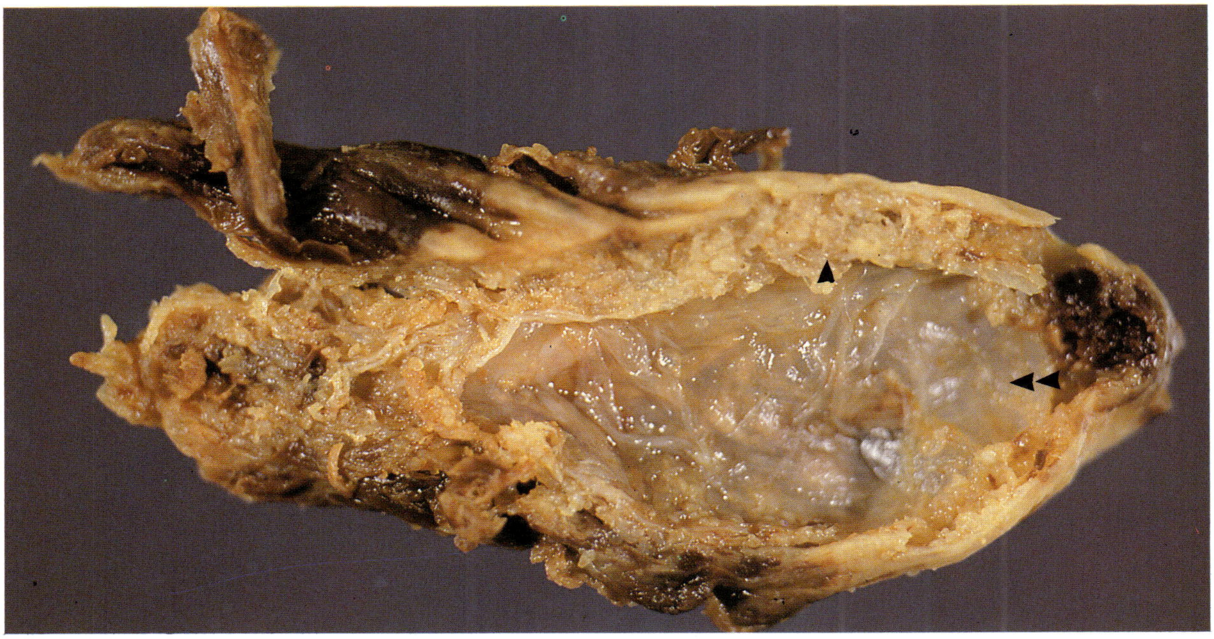

57 A gestational sac passed intact *per vaginam*. The sac has been bisected. No fetal parts were found within it. The chorionic villi (▶) and membranes (▶▶) are obvious in this case but may sometimes be difficult to identify.

58

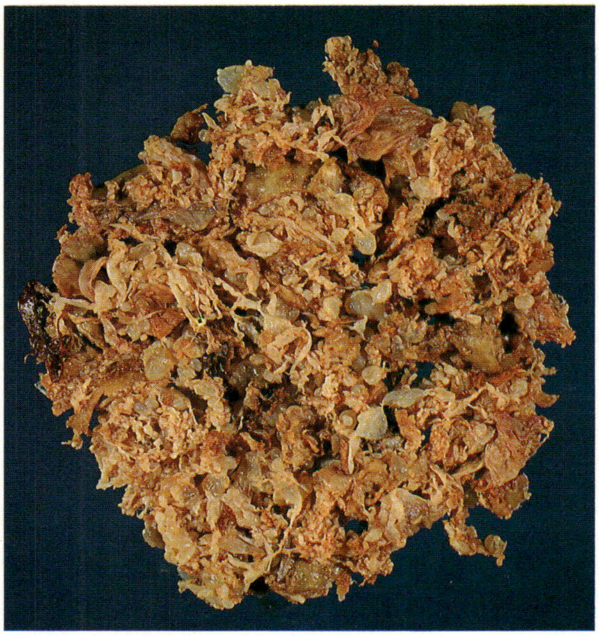

59

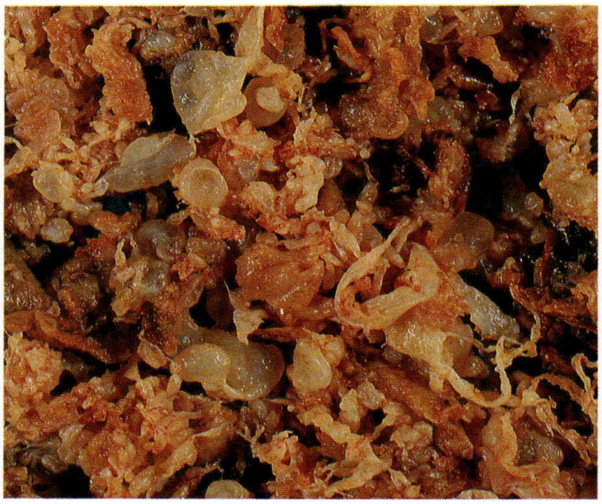

58 Placental tissue from a case of hydatidiform mole. Grape-like chorionic villi can easily be identified in the specimen. Blocks should be taken especially of these.

59 A detail of 58.

60

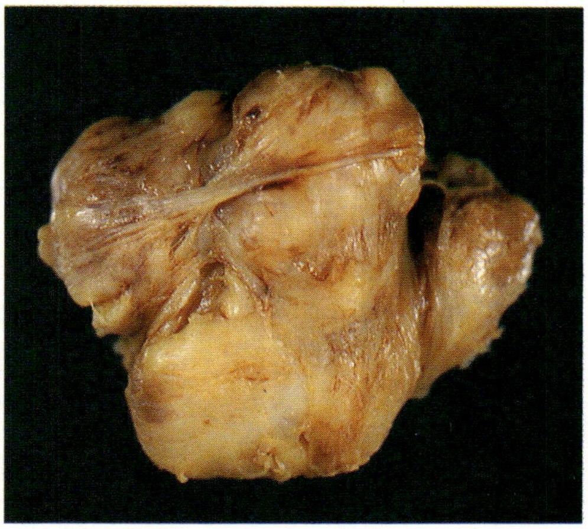

60 An intramural fibroid (leiomyoma) removed by myomectomy. The nodular surface gives the impression that a true capsule is present, but in fact it consists of compressed myometrial fibres around the tumour.

61

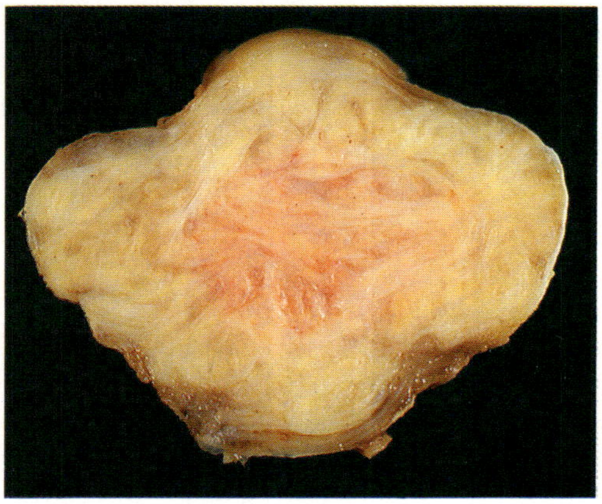

61 The cut surface of 60. The typical whorled pattern of the leiomyoma is apparent.

62 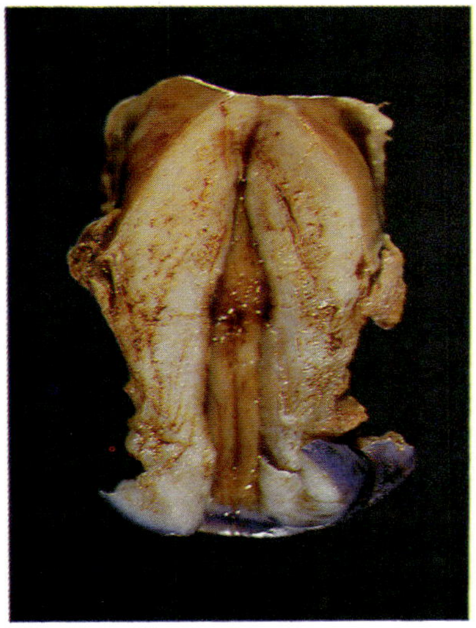

63 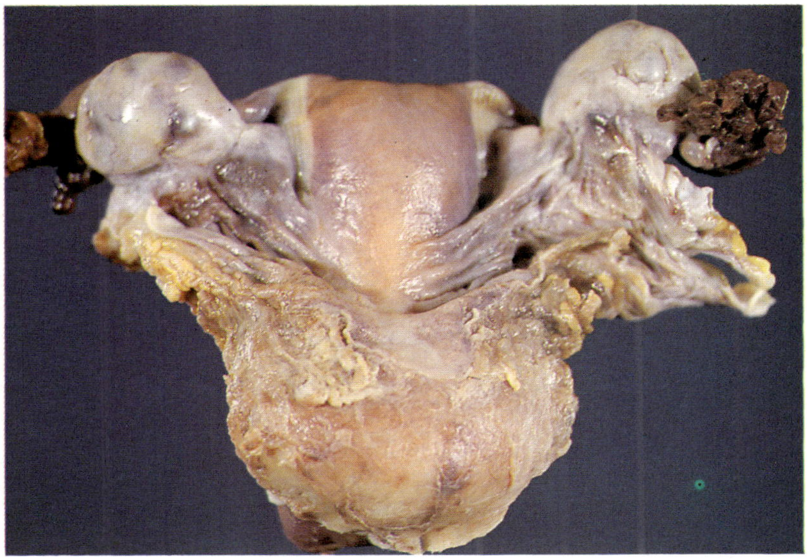

62 A simple hysterectomy specimen. The cervix and vagina were painted with methylene blue by the gynaecologist to help to identify these structures during the operation. The specimen was opened anteriorly in the operating theatre before being immersed in formalin.

63 A radical hysterectomy specimen (posterior aspect) with adjacent parametrium, both ovaries and fallopian tubes, and a cuff of vagina. The operation was performed for cervical carcinoma. The peritoneum over the corpus extends down towards the cervix, further than in the anterior view.

64 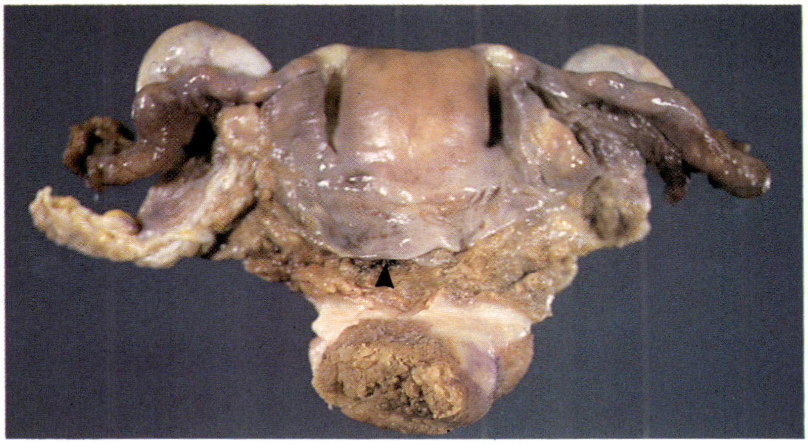

64 The anterior aspect of 63 after removal of the vaginal cuff. The peritoneum covers the upper part of the corpus and is then reflected anteriorly over the adipose tissue between the uterus and the bladder (▶). The insertions of the fallopian tubes are posterior to the round ligaments and anterior to the ovaries.

65 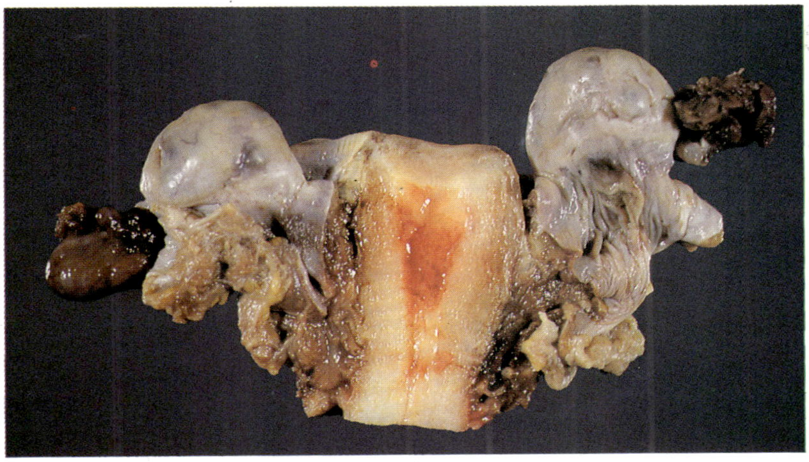

65 The corpus 64 opened along the lateral borders. The resulting tissues consist of the anterior wall of the uterus with attached adnexa (viewed from behind) and the posterior wall (not shown).

66

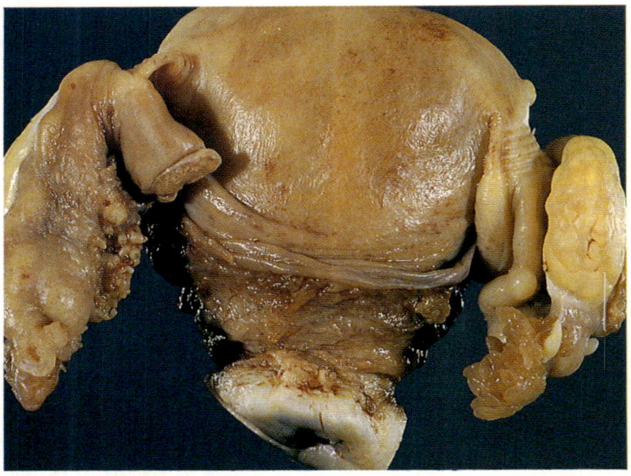

66 A total hysterectomy specimen (anterior aspect) removed for carcinoma of the endometrium.

67a and b The uterus 66 bisected through the lateral borders, leaving the adnexa attached to the anterior half. In the uterine cavity, a soft papillary tumour mass extends into the inner two thirds of the myometrium on the left (▶).

67a

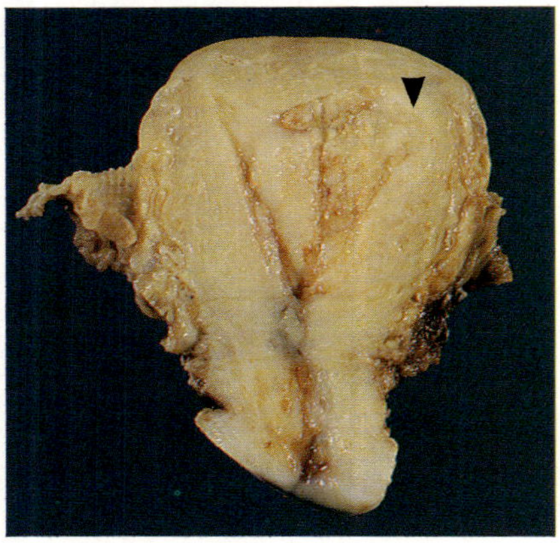

67b

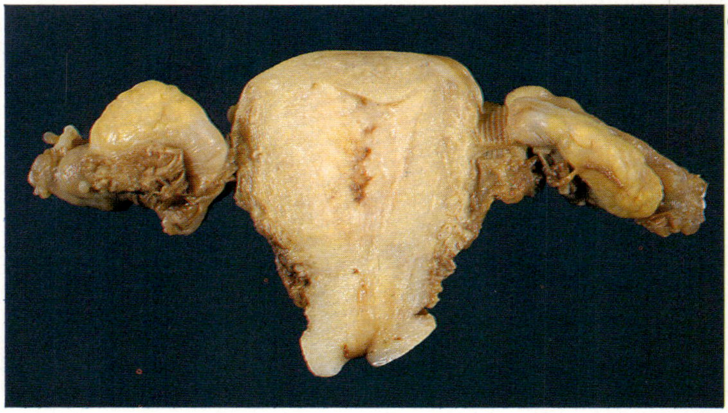

67c

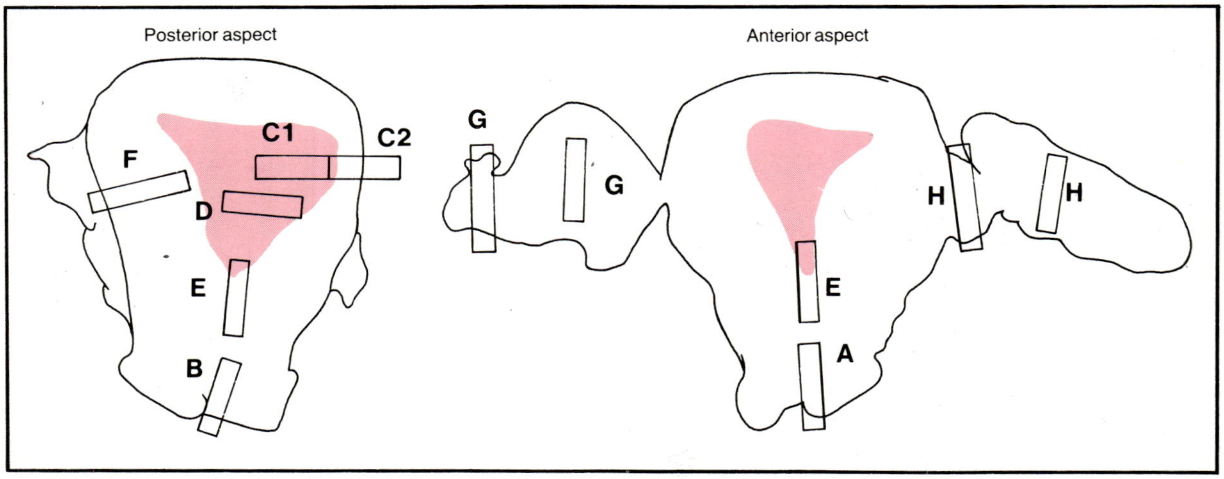

67c Blocks taken from a total hysterectomy for endometrial carcinoma: anterior cervix (**A**); posterior cervix (**B**); tumour and full thickness of uterine wall - endometrial aspect (**C1**); serosal aspect (**C2**); tumour (**D**); tumour and isthmus (**E**); uninvolved endometrium, myometrium and serosa (**F**); right ovary and fallopian tube with parametrium (**G**); left ovary and fallopian tube with parametrium (**H**).

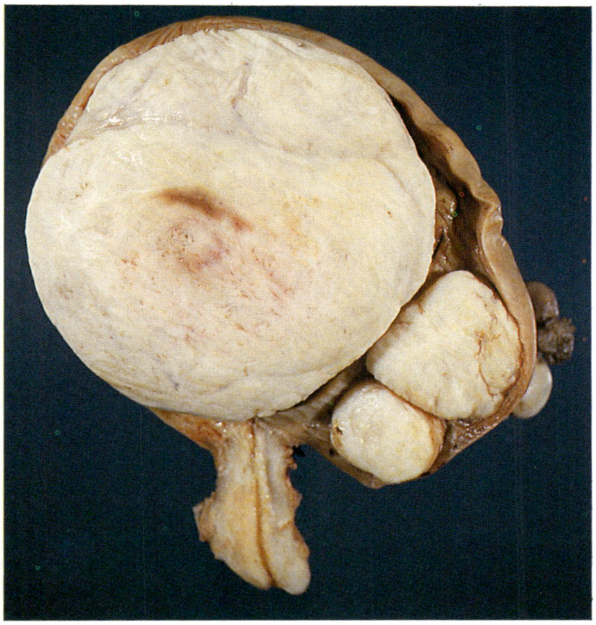

68a A uterus with leiomyomas. There is a large intramural leiomyoma, the centre of which has undergone liquefactive (cystic, pseudocystic) change, and two smaller leiomyomas which have become submucosal and indent the endometrial cavity. The left fallopian tube and ovary are also present. The right adnexa were not excised.

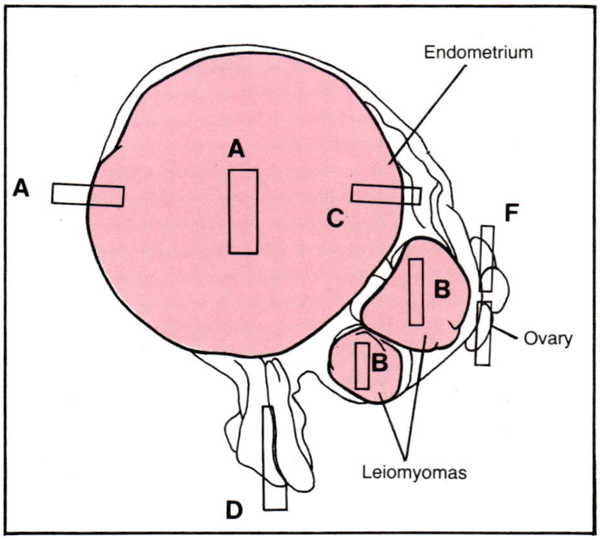

68b Blocks taken from a uterus with leiomyomas: largest leiomyoma (**A**); smaller leiomyomas (**B**); endometrium, uninvolved myometrium and serosa (**C**); anterior cervix (**D**); posterior cervix (**E**—not shown); left fallopian tube and ovary (**F**).

Fallopian tube

Types of specimens

Sterilization procedures

It is important for medicolegal reasons that segments of fallopian tube from sterilization procedures should be sent for histological confirmation. Rarely, a length of round ligament may be excised in error. A short cylinder should be taken from the centre of the specimen and the rest preserved until the case is reported. Usually the left and right tubes are sent separately, and should be blocked separately with the side specified. When only a small segment of tube is excised, orientation with a dissecting microscope may be necessary before the tissue is embedded so that transverse sections can be obtained.

Ectopic pregnancies

Fallopian tubes may be excised in cases of suspected or confirmed tubal pregnancy. These usually show an area of dilatation at the site of the gestation sac or tubal rupture (**69**). Transverse cuts are made through the tube. Blocks should include the blood clot within the tube lumen, where chorionic villi may be found (**70**). Further fixation is often necessary as diffusion of formalin through clot is poor. Blocks should also be taken from the uninvolved tube proximal and distal to the clot. Fibrosis or other pathology in the wall may have led to impairment of ovum transport and therefore to the ectopic gestation. Recognition of this problem is important as the contralateral tube may also be affected.

Salpingitis and other conditions

In specimens removed for salpingitis, endometriosis and other non-neoplastic conditions, several transverse blocks should be taken along the length of the tube. If unfixed material is available, specimens should be sent for microbiological examination.

Carcinoma of fallopian tube

This rare condition is treated surgically as for a malignant ovarian neoplasm, and the specimen should be treated in the same way (p 57).

Fallopian tube: Macroscopical report	
Type of specimen	Sterilization excision specimen, unilateral salpingectomy, salpingo-oophorectomy
Measurements	Length and maximum diameter of specimen
Description	
Serosa	Colour; contour (fusiform swelling at isthmus, in centre or at fimbrial end, dilatation, parovarian cysts on serosa, scarring); texture (fibrinous exudate on serosa, perforation of ectopic gestation)
Wall	Appearance of wall (thickened, thin and attenuated, focally scarred)
Mucosa and contents	Colour; consistency (soft and friable, firm); contents (thin straw-coloured fluid, blood-stained, frank blood, pus, gestational sac, fetal tissues)

69

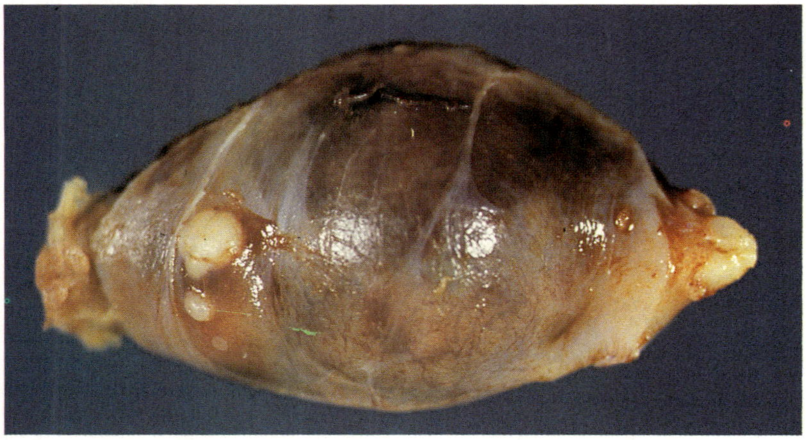

69 A fallopian tube containing an ectopic gestation. The tube is fusiform and plum-coloured, and the serosal vessels are prominent.

70

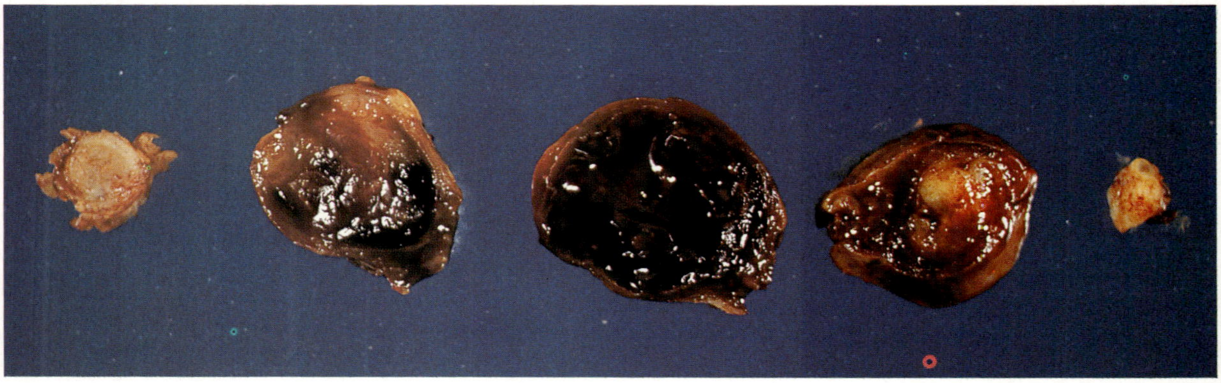

70 Cross sections of the fallopian tube in 69. Fresh blood and clot are apparent but placental and fetal tissue are hard to identify, and numerous blocks will therefore be necessary. The isthmic end of the tube is also examined, to look for fibrosis or other lesions that might have led to the ectopic gestation.

Ovary

Small specimens

The ovary may be biopsied in cases of premature menopause, polycystic ovary syndrome (Stein-Leventhal syndrome) and infertility. Orientation is seldom a problem. The tissue should be blocked whole, or bisected through the long axis perpendicular to the ovarian surface if the specimen is too large to fit into the processing cassette. Description in most cases can be confined to the colour, shape, size and cut surface appearance.

Large specimens

Unilateral oophorectomy is performed for benign ovarian tumours and torsion (**71, 72**). Bilateral removal may be undertaken for palliation of breast carcinoma and, together with hysterectomy, in cases of malignant neoplasms of the female genital tract proximal to the vulva (**73, 74**). The ovaries may sometimes be removed with the hysterectomy specimen in cases of dysfunctional uterine bleeding in patients over the age of 40 years.

Initial dissection

The specimen should be weighed and measured prior to cutting, before the escape of contents and distortion by the collapse of cysts. The contents of cystic ovarian neoplasms may be under pressure, and care must therefore be taken when they are incised.

The consistency of the contents of an ovarian cyst must also be recorded. The consistency may suggest whether the cyst is serous or mucinous, though it is not an infallible guide. On the other hand, sebaceous material nearly always indicates a teratoma. In unilocular and multilocular cysts, the wall should be examined for areas of thickening or irregularity and blocks taken from these. The serosal surface should be examined and blocks taken from roughened, papillary or dull areas. Solid tumours are usually large enough for tissue to be reserved in case fat stains are necessary (**75, 76**).

Blocks should be taken from at least three areas, but with large tumours more will be necessary. The rule of thumb is that one block should be taken for every centimetre of the tumour's diameter, but this would clearly be excessive for large unilocular cysts with smooth uniform walls. Solid areas of tumour should be well sampled, and if possible the capsular surface of the mass should be included, so that its relation with the tumour can be assessed. The staff responsible for section preparation should be warned if it is likely that calcification or bone is present in the blocks.

If the ovary is normal in size, one longitudinal block is usually sufficient. When the fallopian tubes, uterus, cervix and vagina are present, blocks should be taken from them as described above.

Ovary: Macroscopical report	
Type of specimen	Ovarian biopsy, wedge resection, ovarian cystectomy, ovary and fallopian tube, bilateral oophorectomy and salpingectomy (with or without hysterectomy specimen)
Measurements	Weight (useful in large cysts as an indicator of size, and may also be of interest to the patient) Size (diameter if spherical), or range of sizes of cysts
Description	
Outer surface	Smooth, roughened, involved by neoplasm, ruptured, presence of adhesions; capsule (thick, uniform, focally thickened)
Cut section	Cystic (unilocular, multilocular), solid, focally solid, calcification; recognizable tissues (such as hair or teeth); normal structures such as corpora lutea, corpora albicantia
Contents of cysts	Thin, straw-coloured; thick, clear; blood-stained; brown; thick and greasy

Example 73-74

The specimen consists of a uterus and cervix with both adnexa. The right ovary is grossly enlarged; it measures 14.5 × 13 × 12.5 cm and weighs 925 g. The surface is smooth and glistening. The cut surface shows a multiloculated tumour mass. The loculi range from 1-5 cm in diameter, and contain thick clear fluid. No endophytic papillary growth is present in any of the loculi. At one pole of the mass there is a portion of residual ovary, measuring 2 × 1.2 × 1 cm. The cut section shows a corpus luteum. The right fallopian tube is stretched across the ovarian mass, and is 11 cm long with a maximum diameter of 0.8 cm.

The left ovary appears normal, and measures 4 × 1.9 × 1.5 cm. The left fallopian tube is 6 cm long with a uniform diameter of 1.2 cm, and has several parovarian cysts at the fimbrial end.

The uterus and cervix together measure 11 × 6.3 × 5.7 cm and weigh 140 g. The endometrium, myometrium and serosa appear normal. The endocervical canal contains a small mucoid polyp 2 cm long and 0.5 cm in diameter, which protrudes through the external os. The os is slit-shaped and 1.2 cm long. The ectocervix appears macroscopically unremarkable.

Blocks

- A right ovarian tumour × 6
- B right ovary × 2
- C right fallopian tube × 1
- D left ovary × 1
- E left fallopian tube × 2
- F endometrium and myometrium × 2
- G endocervical polyp × 1
- H anterior cervix × 1
- J posterior cervix × 1

71

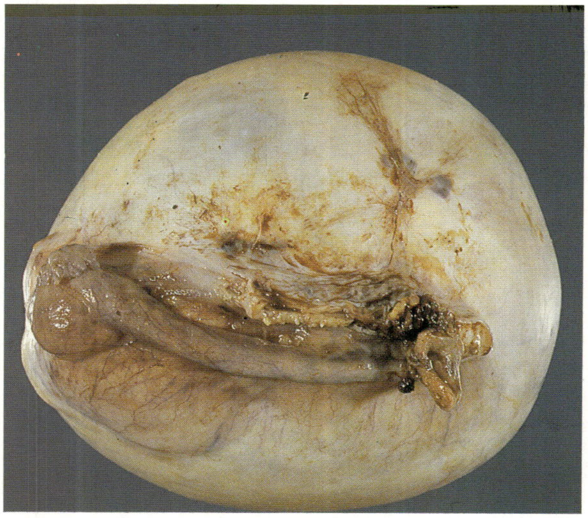

71 A cyst, across which the fallopian tube is stretched (this is in fact a serous cystadenoma, though it is not possible to identify it with certainty from its gross appearances).

72

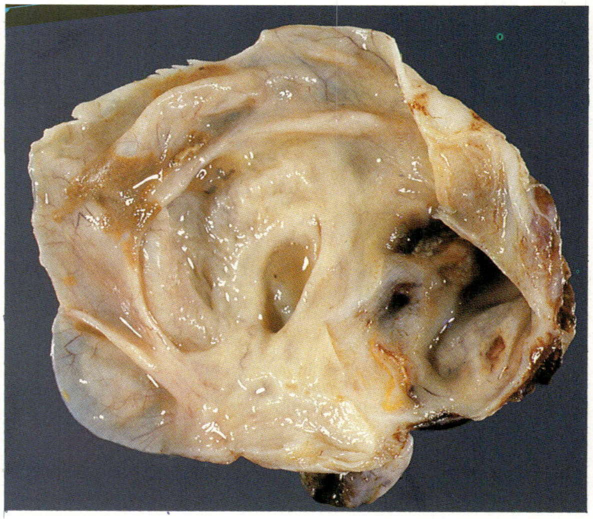

72 Half of the cyst in 71. It has a smooth wall that measures less than 0.2 cm thick and contains clear serous fluid.

73 **A hysterectomy and bilateral salpingo-oophorectomy specimen** for ovarian carcinoma. The right ovary contains a smooth-surfaced cystic mass.

73

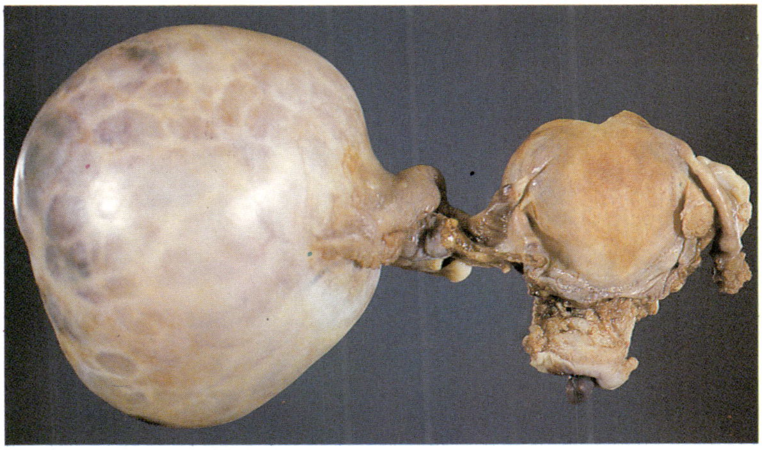

74 **A section of the ovarian cyst in 73.** The lesion is multiloculated, with individual locules ranging in size from 1-5 cm in diameter. Most of them contain clear mucous fluid. On microscopic examination the tumour was found to be a low-grade ('borderline') mucinous cystadenocarcinoma.

74

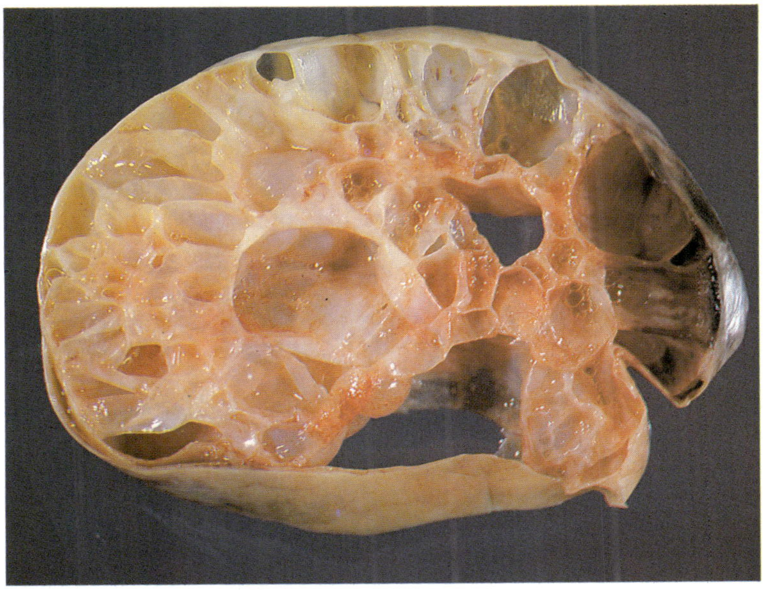

75

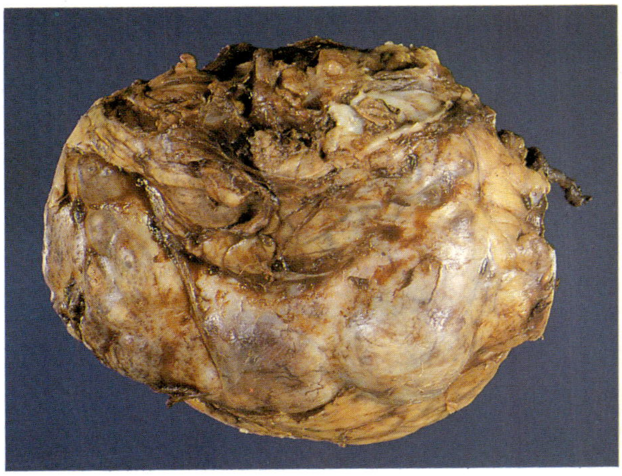

75 **A solid ovarian tumour** with a roughened haemorrhagic surface.

76

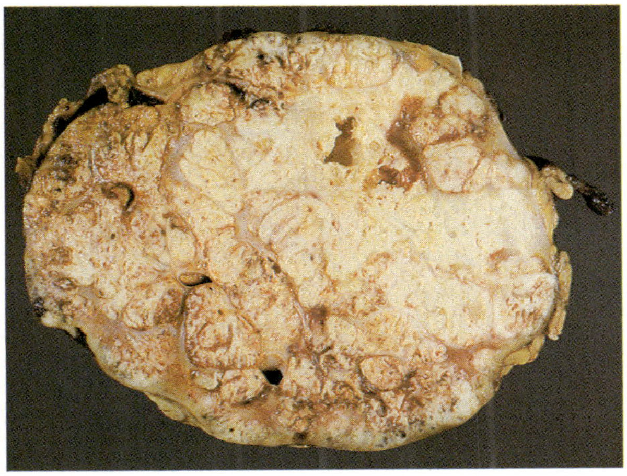

76 **The cut surface of 75.** The tumour is composed of numerous irregular nodules of yellow and white tissue in which there are foci of haemorrhage and necrosis.

Fetus and placenta

Fetus

The method of dissection is determined by the condition of the fetus and its gestational age. The crown-rump, crown-heel and head circumference of the fetus should be measured, but this may be difficult when the fetus has been fixed in a flexed or distorted position (77). Another means of assessing gestational age is foot length (78). Malformed fetuses should be photographed, and radiological examination of all fetuses over about 16 weeks should be performed if possible.

If the fetus is small (less than 10 cm crown-heel length), the external appearances should be recorded and transverse cuts made through the head, thorax and abdomen. These sections can then be examined for congenital abnormalities, using a hand lens or dissecting microscope to check that the major organs are correctly sited and do not have gross congenital abnormalities.

Larger fetuses should be examined externally, and then an internal examination performed as for a necropsy on a full-term infant. Blocks from the heart, both lungs, thymus, adrenals, kidney, liver, spleen, brain, pancreas, gonads, costochondral junction and muscle should be taken if the range of congenital abnormalities is to be investigated in any depth.

Placenta

Placental tissue may be received in small fragments from a spontaneous or therapeutic abortion or retained products of conception. These are considered in the section on uterine corpus (p 48).

Placentas may be sent for histological examination in cases of known or suspected maternal or fetal disease, multiple births, stillbirths, intrauterine infection and small-for-dates babies.

The specimen should be weighed, measured and examined to see whether it is a singleton, twin or multiple placenta (**79-83**) and to check for completeness. Cotyledons or a full succenturiate lobe can be missing, and the only evidence of this may be sheaths of large fetal vessels running across the membranes and ending abruptly. When placentitis (chorioamnionitis) is suspected and fresh tissue is available, a specimen should be sent for microbiological examination. The villi of a hydatidiform mole are usually easily recognizable (**58, 59**).

The placenta should be examined if possible before fixation, starting with the umbilical cord and membranes. The length of the cord and the number of vessels in it should be recorded. The type of insertion (central, submarginal, marginal, velamentous) and the presence of atresia, knots, haemorrhage and inflammation should also be noted. The membranes should be closely inspected, especially in cases of multiple gestation.

With the maternal surface of the placenta upwards, the cotyledons are cut with a long-bladed knife at 2 cm intervals, towards the fetal surface but not through it, so that the membranes keep the slices of placenta in sequence (**84**). Slicing at intervals of less than 2 cm may cause fragmentation. The slices should be examined for areas of necrosis, haemorrhage, oedema, angiomatous malformations and other focal lesions, and the specimen then allowed to fix fully. Alternatively, the cuts can pass through the entire specimen; the slices are then laid out in sequence and fixed separately (**85**).

Blocks should be taken from the central and peripheral parts of the placenta; from both the maternal and fetal aspects; from any focal lesion; from the umbilical cord; and from the membranes (**80b**). A roll can be made of membranes and a short cylinder cut from it for embedding on end (**80b, 84**). In multiple pregnancies, the blocks from the placenta of each infant should be kept separate. Samples of the common membrane(s) should also be taken for histological examination.

77 Fetus, umbilical cord and placenta from a patient who miscarried at 12 weeks.

77

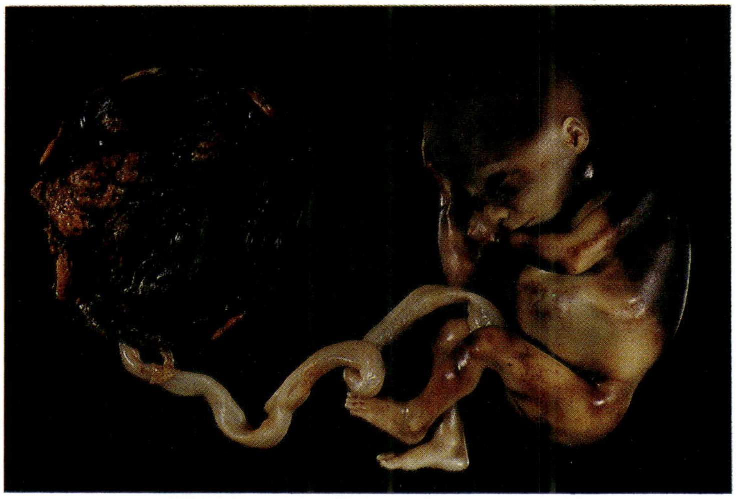

78

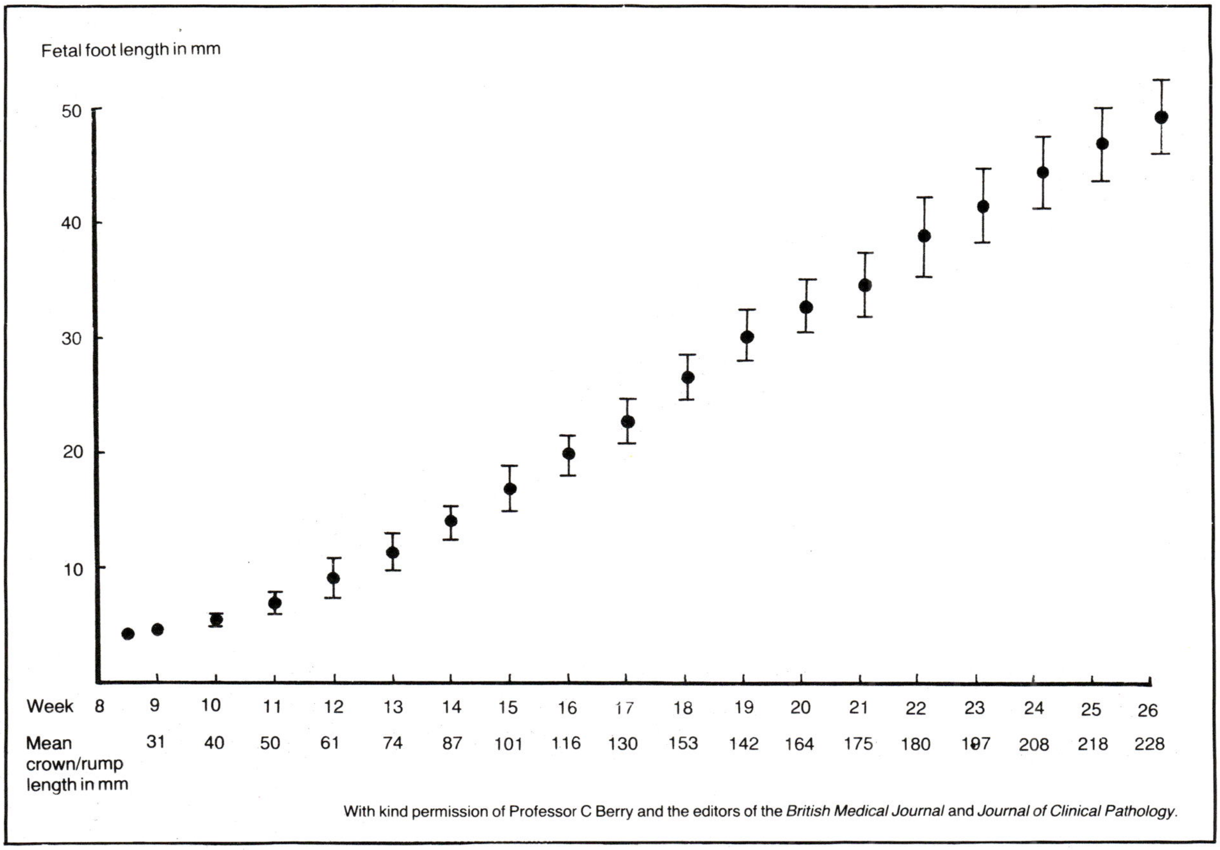

78 Graph showing the relationship between foot length and gestational age.

79

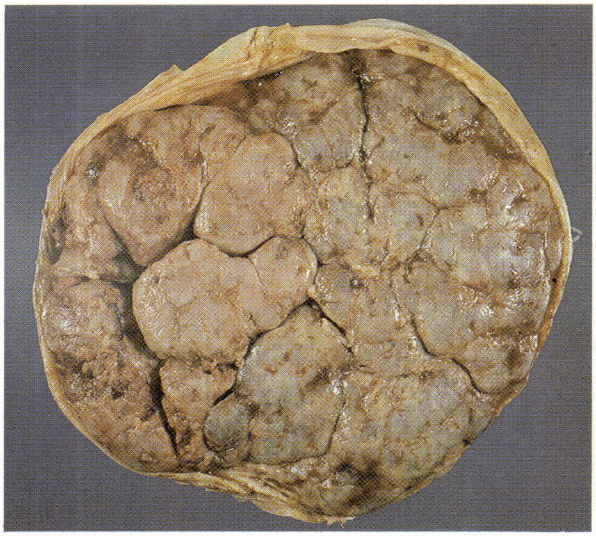

80a

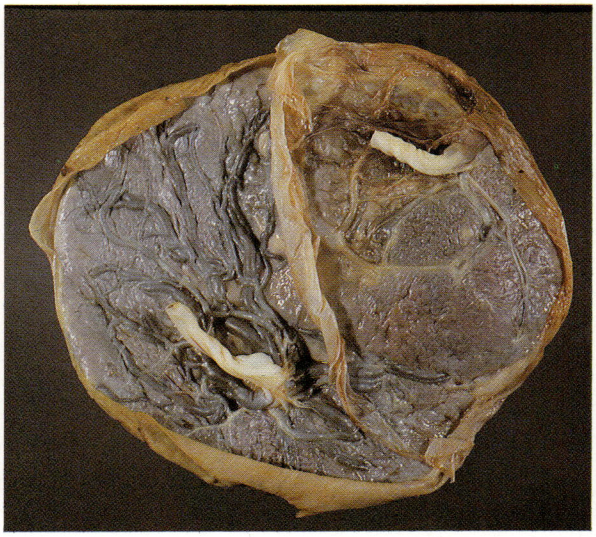

80b

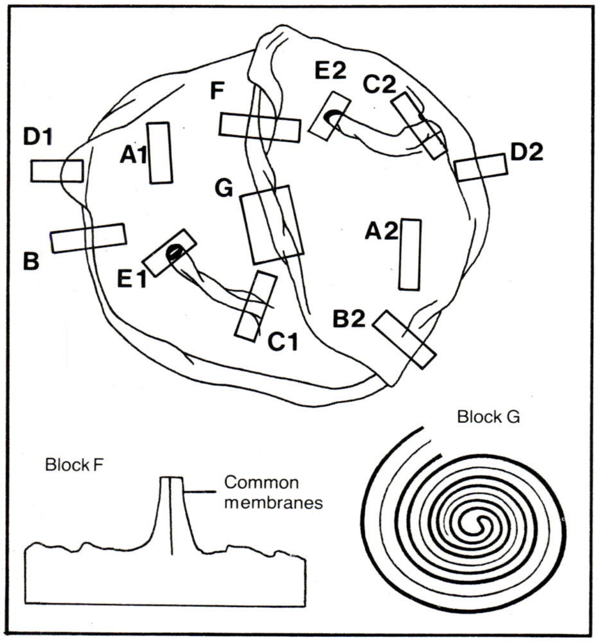

79 Placenta from a twin pregnancy (maternal surface) in which the twin-twin transfusion syndrome had occurred. There is a complete set of cotyledons and no obvious division into separate units. The cotyledons of twin 1 are pale and oedematous (on the left). The part of the placenta supplying twin 2 (on the right) is deep red.

80a The fetal surface of 79. The vessels supplying twin 1 are small and empty (on the right) whereas those supplying twin 2 are dilated and congested.

80b Blocks taken from a twin placenta. Blocks from each twin are kept separate from each other and from the common membrane. Placental blocks are full thickness, including both maternal and fetal surfaces. Central part of placenta (**A1, A2**); peripheral part of placenta (**B1, B2**); placenta below insertion of cord (**C1, C2**); lateral membrane (**D1, D2**); umbilical cord (**E1, E2**); common membrane and underlying placenta (**F**); common membrane (**G**). (Additional blocks should be taken from any focal lesions.)

81

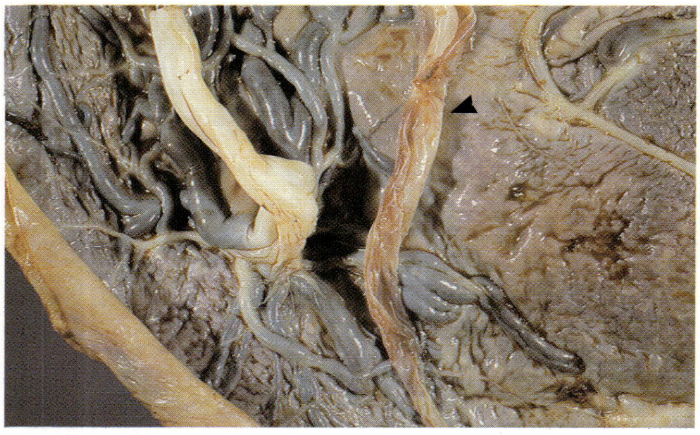

81 Anastomic vessels between the circulations of twin 1 and twin 2. An arrow marks the common membranes.

82

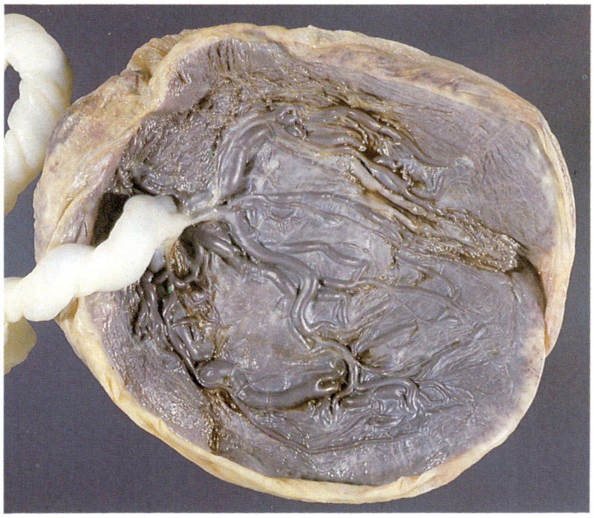

83

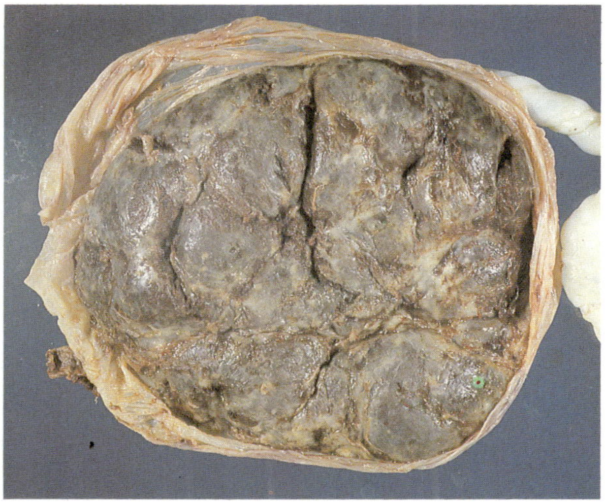

82 and 83 **Fetal** (82) **and maternal** (83) **aspects** of a circummarginate singleton placenta. The umbilical cord is inserted eccentrically.

84

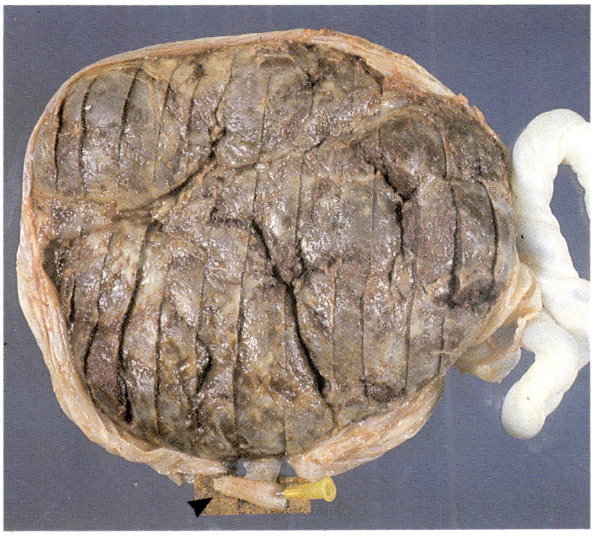

84 The placenta 82 sliced leaving the membranes intact. A roll has been made of membranes and is retained by a pin (▶).

85

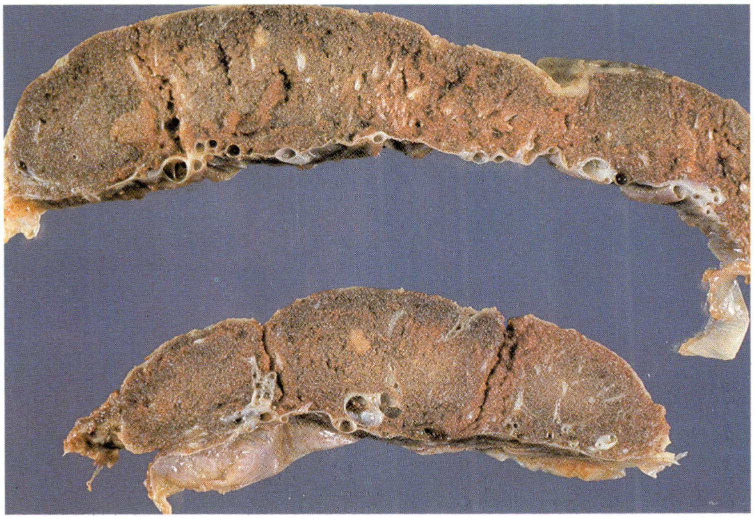

85 Slices through 82, 83. On microscopic examination, the tiny white patches were found to be areas of intervillous fibrin deposition.

CHAPTER 4
BREAST

Biopsies

Biopsies are often taken from the breast to diagnose the cause of palpable lumps, bleeding from the nipple and, increasingly, from areas of microcalcification found by screening mammography. These may be drill or needle biopsies, or incisional or excisional biopsies (**86, 87**). The latter may be sent with axillary contents.

Orientation of most needle or small biopsies is not important and in fact is usually impossible. The specimen is briefly described and embedded whole.

Larger biopsies in which a focal lesion is palpable are cut into thin parallel slices to reveal the pathology present (**86**). For excisional biopsies the outer surface should be marked with India ink before slicing or blocking, so that the proximity of a tumour to the excision lines may be assessed easily. Blocks are taken from focal lesions and the tissues adjacent to them, areas of calcification and excision margins.

Guide wire biopsies, performed to excise suspicious non-palpable lesions revealed by mammography, require special handling by the pathologist. The whole specimen should be X-rayed before any dissection to ensure that the abnormality seen radiographically in the patient has in fact been removed (**88**). The specimen is then cut into parallel sagittal slices not more than 0.5 cm thick, and these are laid out in numbered sequence. (Orientation is usually only possible if the surgeon has marked some aspect of the biopsy with a suture.) Keeping the slices in order, the entire specimen is then X-rayed again (**89**). In some departments the above procedure is carried out before fixation so that areas with radiographic appearances suspicious of carcinoma can be sampled for oestrogen receptor analysis, if the amount of tissue permits. After fixation, all areas showing microcalcification are submitted for histological examination by dividing the slices into blocks of appropriate size. It is important to ink the excision margins before histological processing so that if carcinoma is found, adequacy of excision be assessed accurately. Other pigments can also be used (p9).

When specimen radiography is not possible, all the tissue around a guide wire should be submitted. If axillary contents are received they are treated as for mastectomy specimens (see below).

Whole specimen radiography should also

Breast biopsies: Macroscopical report	
Site	Right or left breast Position in breast (subareolar, upper outer quadrant etc)
Type of specimen	Drill or needle biopsy, incisional biopsy, excision biopsy, axillary fat and lymph nodes
Measurements	Size of the specimen Size of any focal lesion
Description	
Focal lesions	Colour (uniform white, grey with yellow flecks); contour (irregular, rounded and circumscribed, infiltrating); consistency (rubbery, gritty, hard)
Rest of specimen	Presence of cysts, fibrosis, distended ducts

be undertaken on non-guide wire biopsies if no focal lesion is palpable and there is clinical or cytological suspicion of cancer. If abnormalities are apparent on this X-ray, the specimen should be handled as for a guide wire biopsy. If no radiographic lesion is seen the biopsy is cut into thin parallel slices after fixation. Areas with different gross appearances should be thoroughly sampled.

The dissection of subareolar wedge resections thought clinically to contain duct papillomas is described below in the section on large specimens.

Large specimens

Large specimens from the breast comprise subareolar resection specimens, wedge resections and segmental mastectomy (**90**), simple and extended mastectomies (with or without axillary contents) (**94, 98**), and subcutaneous mastectomies. Radical mastectomies include breast, pectoral muscles, axillary contents, internal mammary and other lymph nodes, but this operation is seldom performed nowadays. Malignant disease is by far the commonest reason for mastectomy. Smaller amounts of tissue may occasionally be excised for the treatment of duct papilloma (**101, 102**), cosmetic breast reduction or gynaecomastia.

Initial dissection

On receipt, the breast resection specimens should be measured. The weight is also useful in operations for breast reduction, in order to assess the symmetry of the operation. Unless axillary contents are attached to the specimen or the surgeon has inserted a suture marker, orientation may not be possible.

The breast tissue should be palpated to identify a focal lesion such as a carcinoma, and a single cut made through it (**91**). Where orientation is possible, the cut should be sagittal; where it is not, the cut should be at right angles to the longest axis of the specimen. If there is skin attached to the specimen, the cut is made into the posterior aspect of the breast as far as the overlying dermis, by placing the specimen epidermis-downwards on the cutting board and using a long-bladed knife. This procedure demonstrates the relation of the tumour to the deep and lateral excision margins and, where applicable, these can then be painted with India ink (**92**). The highest extension of the axillary contents should also be marked so that on later dissection the position of any lymph nodes can be identified.

In some departments, assay for oestrogen receptors will be required, and the specimen will arrive chilled and unfixed. After the initial incision has been made, small cubes of tissue are taken from the fresh tumour and frozen in liquid nitrogen or isopentane/dry ice as soon as possible.

Several cuts at about 1-1.5 cm intervals should then be made parallel to the initial incision leaving the dermis and epidermis intact. The breast slices thus remain in sequence, 'hinged' on the intact skin ellipse (**92**), and can be palpated to search for small lesions less than 1 cm in diameter. Sheets of absorbent paper may be inserted between the leaves of the tissue to aid fixation (**99**). Alternatively, the breast slices may be separated and laid out in sequence (**93, 95, 96, 97**). Where a focal lesion has not been identified, similar parallel cuts are made.

Subareolar wedge resections and other specimens for intraductal lesions below the nipple are uncommon and should, if possible, be sent fresh to the laboratory. Diagnosis of an intraduct papilloma or papillary carcinoma is greatly facilitated by opening the specimen with fine scissors along the affected large duct and pinning out onto a cork board, so that the tumour can be properly fixed and orientated (**101, 102**). If no duct can be identified, the specimen should be left whole until fixed.

Dissection of specimen

After fixation, the component parts of the specimen should be measured, if this has not already been done. Measurements of breast carcinomas have important management implications and should be in millimetres. In some departments, radiography of the breast slices is performed to provide correlation with mammograms and to indicate specific areas from which blocks should be taken.

The axillary tissue and upper outer quadrant of the breast should be palpated and dissected to look for lymph nodes. The proximal and distal groups of axillary nodes are blocked separately. The sliced breast should be examined to establish the macroscopical features of the tumour and its extent of spread. The nipple should be inspected for evidence of Paget's disease or direct involvement of the nipple stroma by underlying carcinoma. Blocks are then taken from the tumour, the deep resection line, and the breast away from the tumour (**94b, 96b, 97b**). The number of blocks taken from the nipple and skin overlying the tumour will depend upon the gross appearance (**103**). Where there has been a previous biopsy, the cavity in the subsequent mastectomy should be extensively sampled to look for residual tumour (**96b**).

Wedge resections and segmental mastectomies can seldom be orientated with confidence unless the surgeon has marked a particular aspect with a suture or other marker. They should be handled as described above.

In a subareolar resection specimen, an intraduct tumour and its stalk (**101, 102**) should not be cut unless it is too large to be embedded whole. Distortion may occur making assessment of invasion difficult. Blocks of the tumour and underlying tissues, the adjacent and other large ducts and of the breast away from the lesion should be submitted. Where no large ducts have been identified in the unfixed specimen, the tissue is cut at close intervals and numerous blocks submitted.

Breast resection specimens: Macroscopical report

Type of specimen	Subareolar resection, wedge resection (segmental mastectomy), simple mastectomy, extended mastectomy, subcutaneous mastectomy, radical mastectomy
Measurements	Weight of the specimen if relevant Maximum and minimum dimensions of the skin ellipse Diameter and thickness of the disc of breast tissue below the skin Dimensions of the axillary tail, if present
Description	
Focal lesion	Site in relation to the standard quadrants of the breast (upper, outer, upper inner, subareolar, etc.) Size in millimetres Colour; consistency (rubbery, hard, gritty, soft, friable, blood-filled cavity); contour (indistinct, extensively infiltrating, circumscribed) Relation of the tumour with the deep and lateral excision lines and with other tissues (muscle, fascia, skin) which may be present
Breast skin	Colour; texture (excoriated, shiny); contour (dimpled, smooth); consistency (oedematous, fibrosed)
Nipple	Excoriated, indurated, inverted or erythematous, directly involved by subareolar tumour
Lymph nodes	Number, sizes, and appearance of lymph nodes, especially in the axillary tail of the specimen

Example 94-97

The specimen is an extended mastectomy consisting of an ellipse of nipple-bearing skin measuring 17 × 8 cm with a disc of underlying breast tissue measuring 22.5 × 17 × 7 cm. Axillary adipose tissue measuring 8.5 × 7 × 2.5 cm is attached to the upper outer quadrant. The skin lateral to the nipple shows an area of bruising 2.7 cm in diameter, and there is tethering of the skin to an underlying lesion. Sections through this show a well-circumscribed cavity 2.5 cm in diameter containing blood clot. In the medial wall of the cavity there is a firm gritty mass with ill-defined edges, measuring 14 × 21 × 22 mm. This is well clear of the deep and lateral excision margins. There is no evidence of direct invasion of the overlying skin or nipple.

The rest of the breast shows no macroscopical abnormality. In the axillary extension, four lymph nodes are found in the distal portion and eight in the proximal part.

Blocks

A	apical axillary lymph node × 1
B	distal axillary lymph nodes × 8
C	proximal axillary lymph nodes × 4
D	tumour × 2
E	biopsy site × 3
F	deep resection margin × 2
G	nipple × 2
H-L	breast away from tumour, superolateral, superomedial, inferolateral and inferomedial quadrants × 1 each

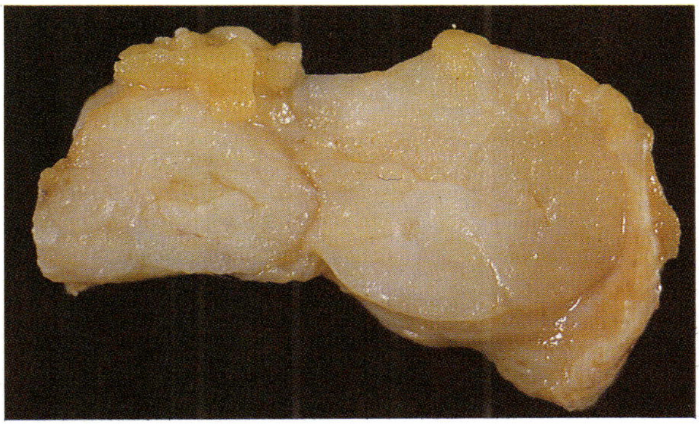

86

86 The cut surface of a fibroadenoma, showing the typical white, circumscribed, lobulated appearance.

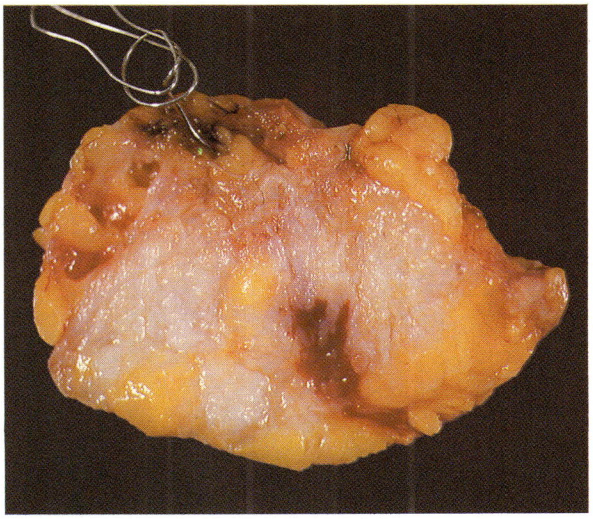

87

87 A guide wire biopsy of the breast with the wire still *in situ*.

88

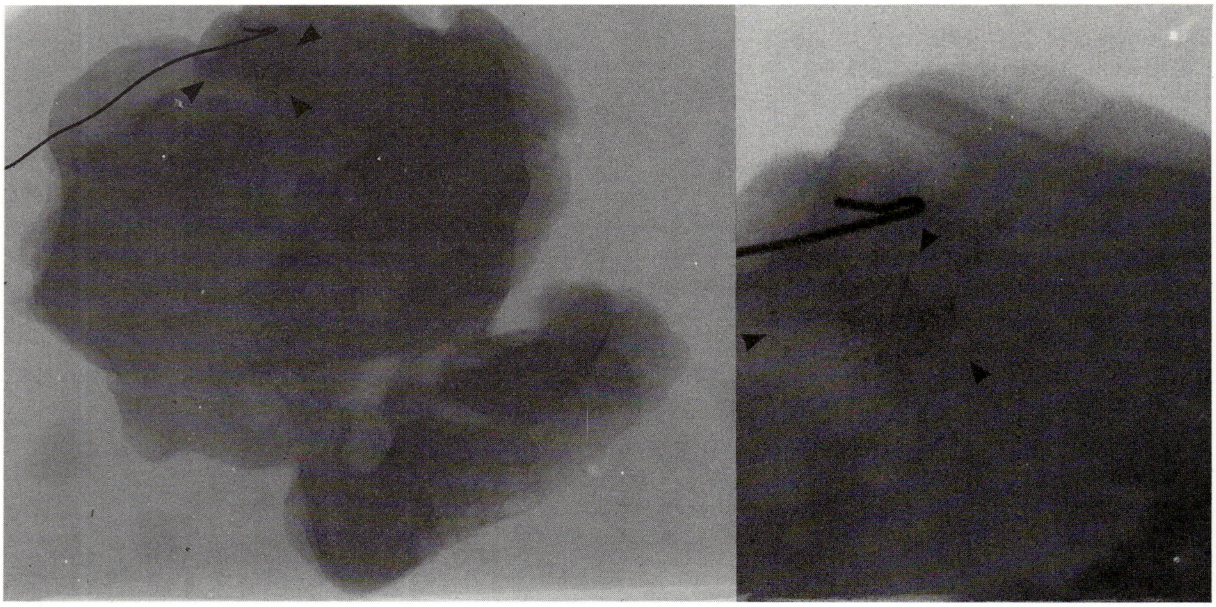

89

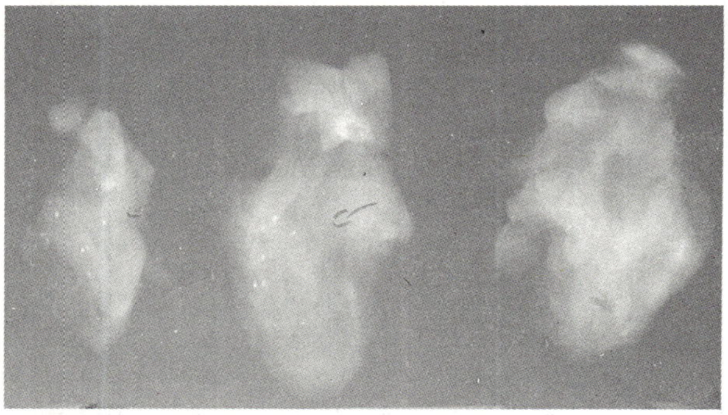

88 Radiograph of a guide wire breast biopsy. Microcalcification can clearly be seen as tiny foci of dense white stippling adjacent to the tip of the wire (▶).

89 X-ray of thin slices of 88.

90

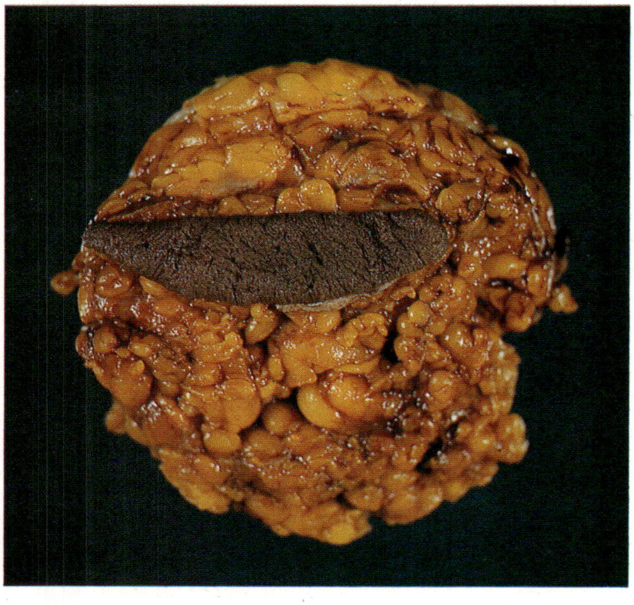

90 A segmental mastectomy specimen with a narrow ellipse of overlying darkly pigmented skin. No nipple is present.

91 Specimen 90 showing the initial cut into the tumour through the posterior surface of the breast to take tissue for oestrogen receptors.

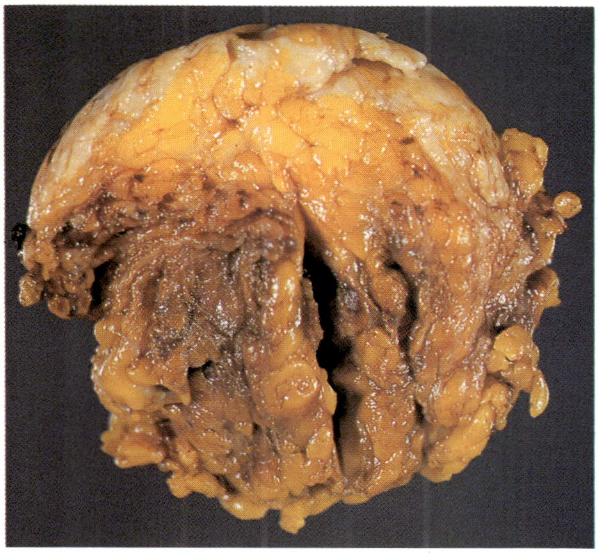

91

92 Specimen 90. Further cuts have been made through the breast parallel to the first incision, and left attached by the skin ellipse to keep them in sequence. The tissue is then allowed to fix further. The tumour was found to be close to the deep resection line, and this has been inked in the centre of the specimen.

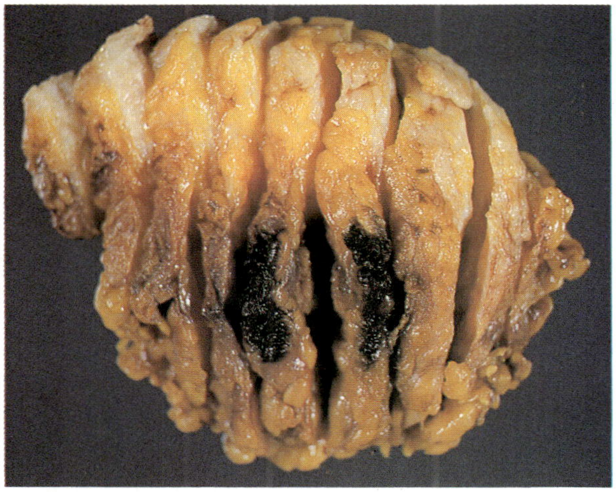

92

93 Specimen 90. As an alternative method, the slices can be separated, laid out in a tray in sequence, and allowed to fix. An ill-defined area of soft tumour tissue can be seen in the centre of one slice (▶). The dense white tissue is an area of fibrosis.

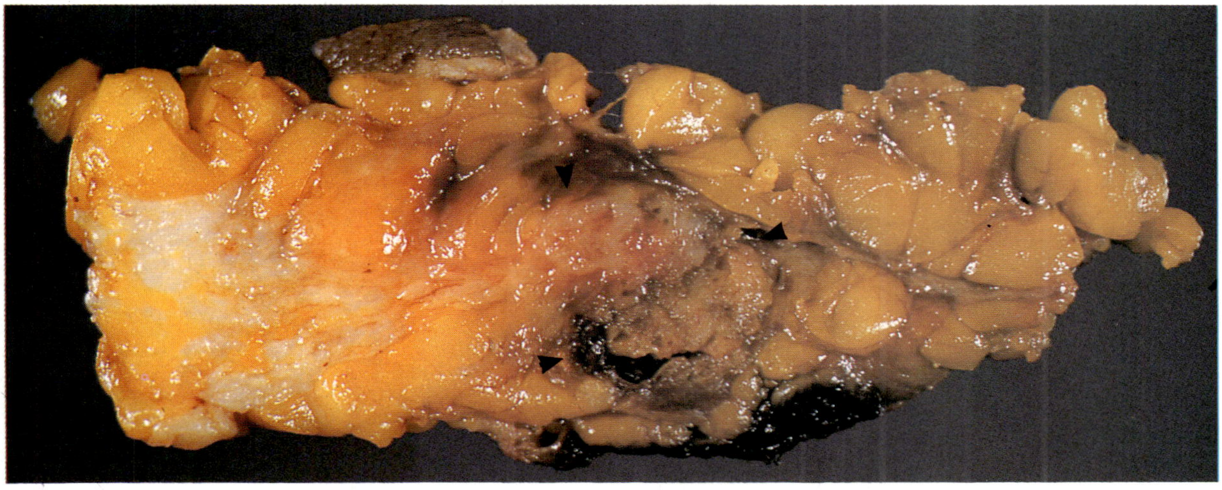

93

94a

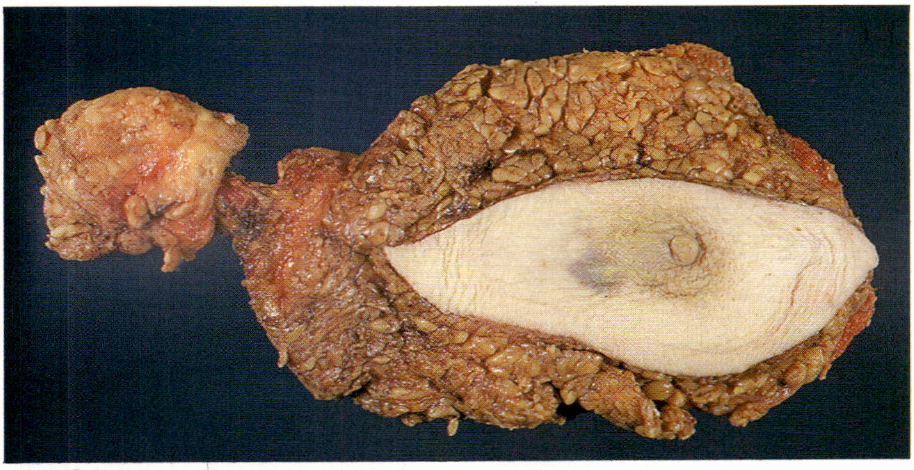

94b

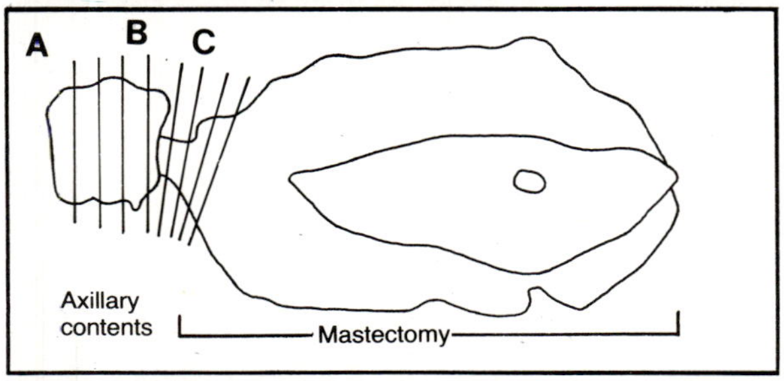

94a An extended mastectomy specimen. There is an ellipse of pale nipple-bearing skin overlying an ovoid mass of breast tissue with an axillary extension to the left containing enlarged lymph nodes. The site of a previous biopsy can be seen lateral to the nipple.

94b Mastectomy specimen blocks, Part 1 (for Part 2, see **96b**). If there is attached axillary fat, this is examined for lymph nodes. The apical (**A**), distal (**B**), and proximal (**C**) nodes (relative to the breast) should be embedded separately.

95

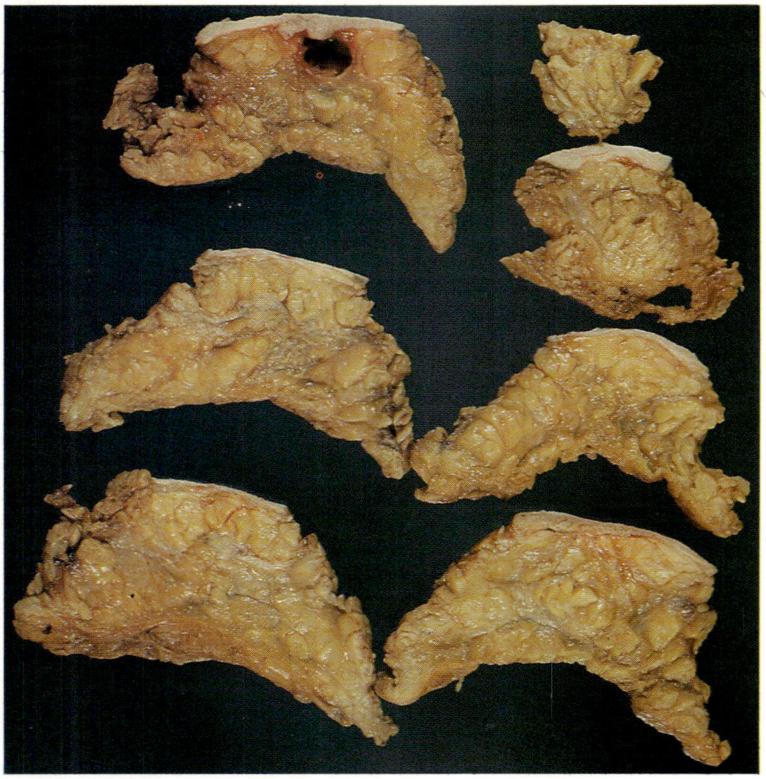

95 Parallel cuts in specimen 94. The cuts have been made through the posterior aspect of the specimen, and the slices laid out in sequence for fixation.

96a A slice of specimen 94 showing the site of the small volume of tissue sent for frozen section diagnosis (▶). Even if no tumour is visible macroscopically, several blocks should be taken from this area.

96a

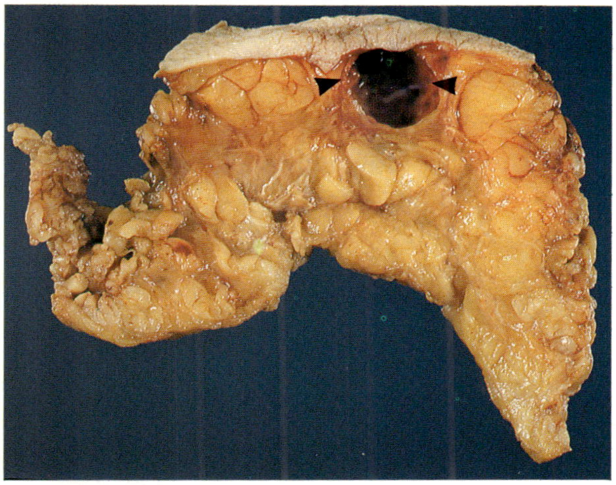

97a The slice adjacent to 96a. Residual tumour is present (▶).

97a

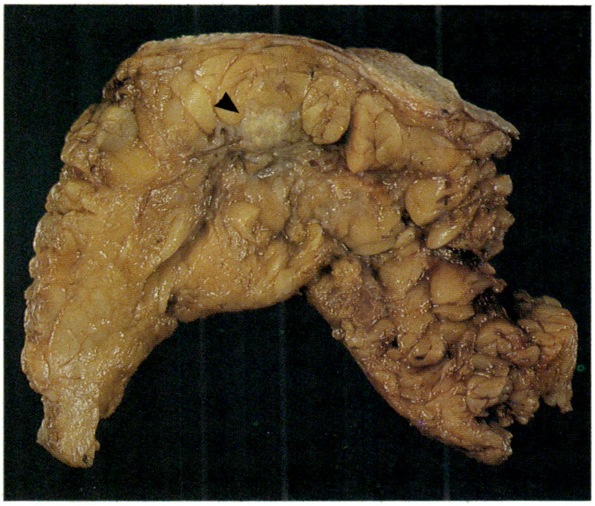

96b and 97b Blocks taken from a mastectomy specimen, Parts 2 and 3: tumour (**D**); biopsy site (**E**); deep excision margin (**F**); nipple (**G**); breast away from tumour (**H, J, K, L**), blocks from the 4 quadrants (**K** and **L** not shown).

96b 97b

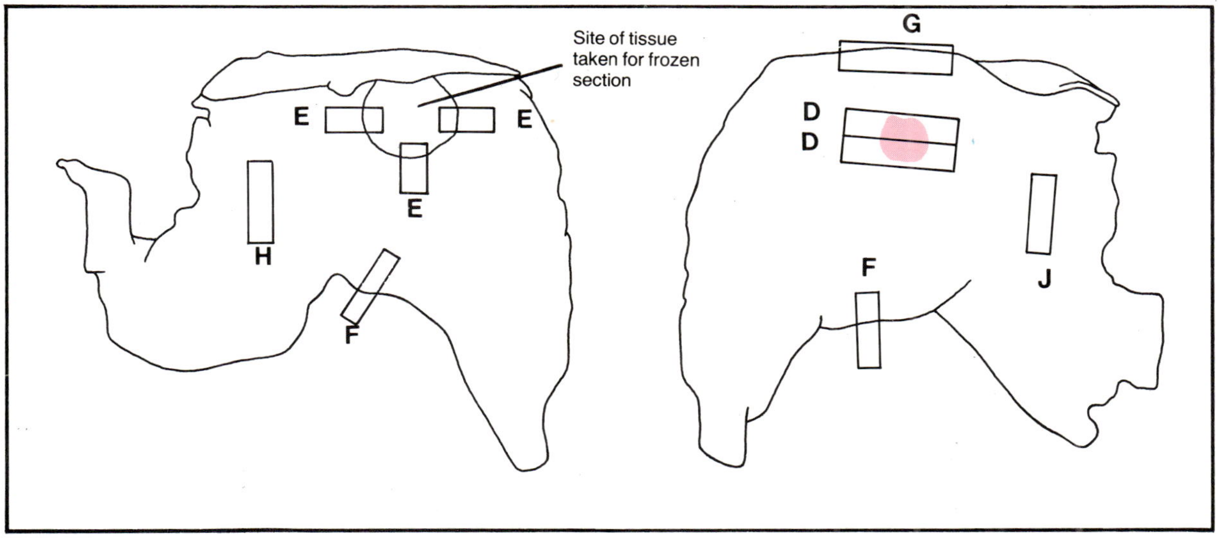

98

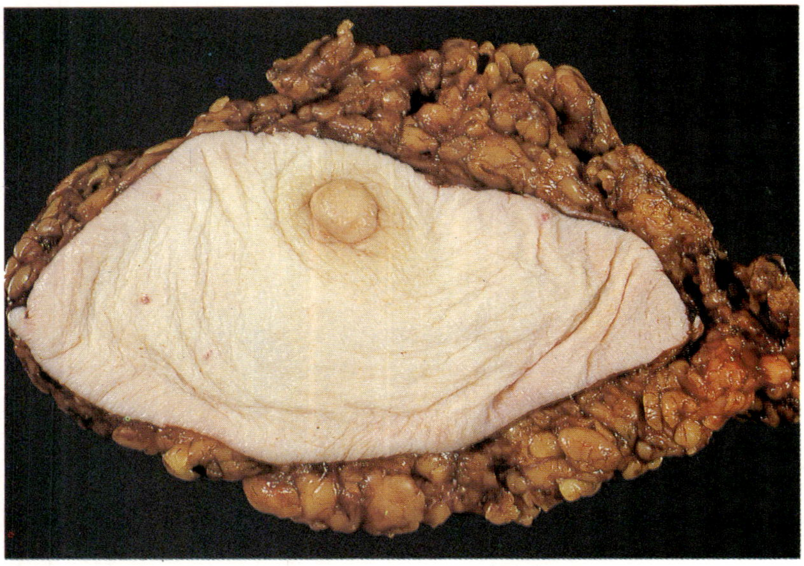

98 A simple mastectomy specimen, consisting of an ellipse of pale nipple-bearing skin overlying a disc of adipose breast tissue.

99

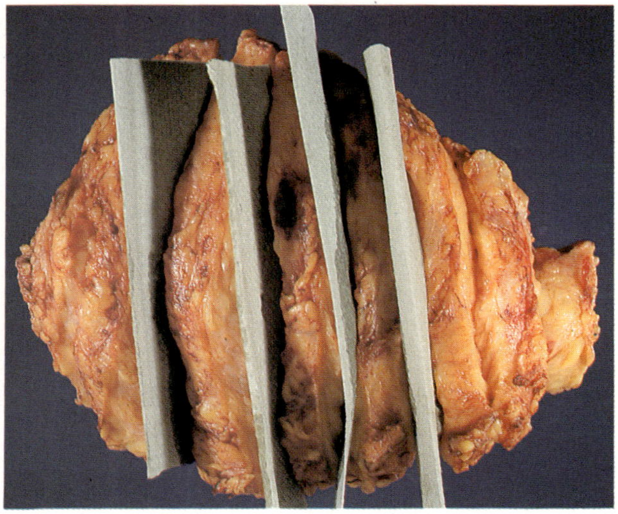

99 Cuts in specimen 98. Absorbent paper can be inserted into the cuts to aid fixation.

100

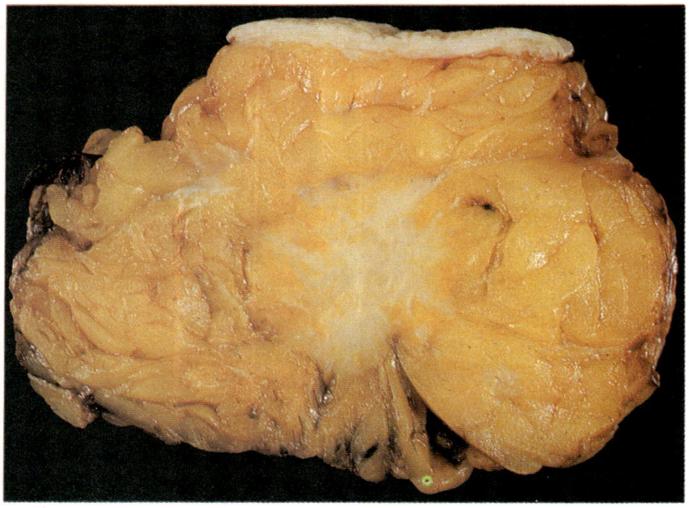

100 The cut surface of a slice from 98 showing a typical scirrhous breast carcinoma.

101 An excision biopsy of the breast containing a relatively large intraduct papilloma. The main ducts have been opened and the tissue pinned out to fix.

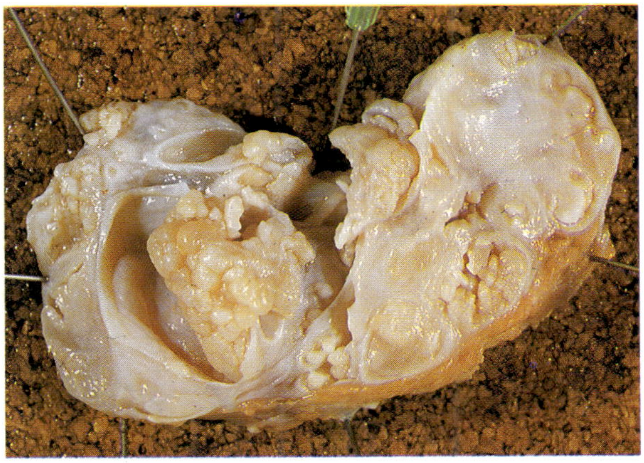
101

102 A close-up view of 101 showing the multinodular papillomatous mass within a cystically dilated duct.

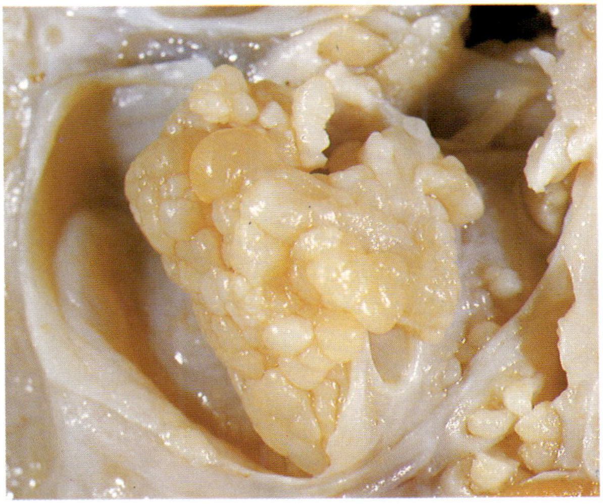
102

103 Dissection of the nipple. Method 1 Parallel sagittal cuts are made through the nipple, and one or more slices embedded. **Method 2** Coronal cuts are made through the nipple and all the tissue embedded (**A-C**). Radial cuts are then made in the areola and associated soft tissue containing the lower parts of the large lacteriferous ducts. The number of blocks embedded will depend on the macroscopical features present.

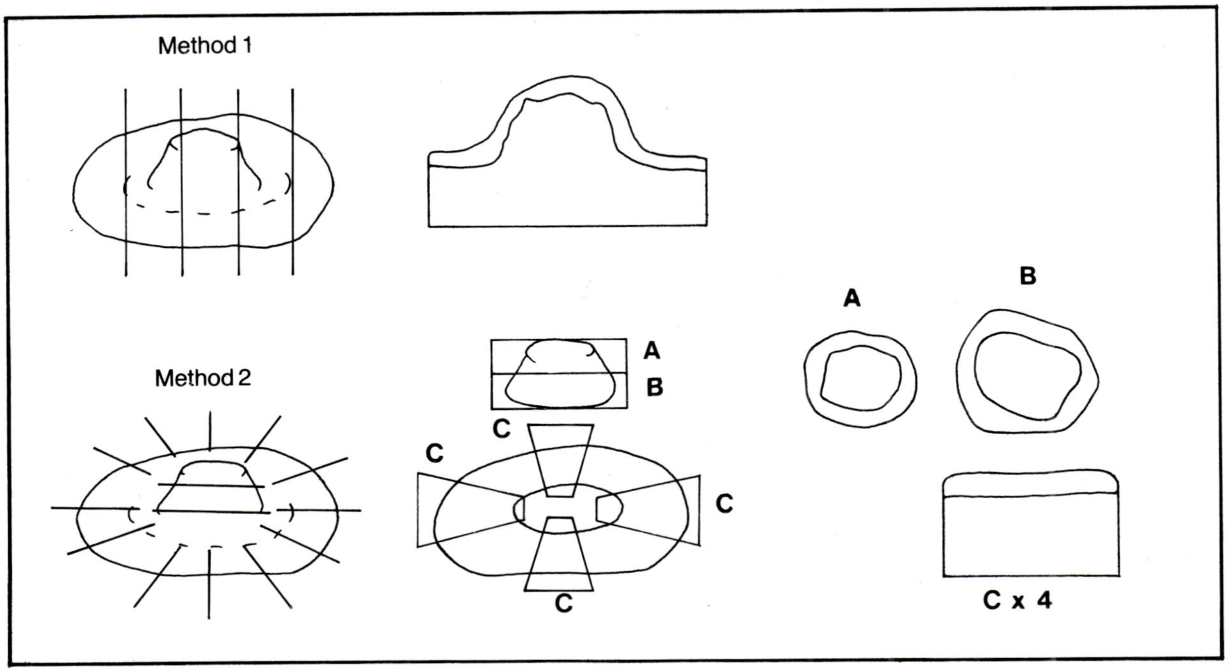

103

CHAPTER 5
MALE GENITAL SYSTEM

Testis

Small specimens

Testicular biopsies for the investigation of infertility should be fixed as soon as possible after excision using Bouin's fixative rather than formalin. This preserves fine cellular detail, tubular architecture, Reinke crystalloids in Leydig cells and in particular the morphology of Sertoli cell nuclei so that it is easier to distinguish them from spermatogonia. If there is likely to be any delay in processing, however, Bouin's-fixed specimens should be transferred to formalin after about an hour to prevent the tissue becoming hard and difficult to section. Small 'keyhole' biopsies, where the testis is not fully exposed and the biopsy is taken through a very small incision, should be discouraged because of the distortion which can result.

Orientation of these small specimens is seldom possible. The tissue is usually measured, described simply (e.g. 'An irregular pale fragment measuring . . .') and embedded whole.

Large specimens

Orchiectomy may be performed for several reasons, including maldescent, torsion, tumour, palliation of a prostatic adeno-carcinoma or as a necessary manoeuvre at herniorrhaphy. Occasionally, cases of orchitis can mimic carcinoma and necessitate orchidectomy.

Dissection of specimen

Bouin's fixative should not be used for orchiectomy specimens as rapid fixation of the outer portions would prevent penetration of the fixative to the centre. Testes may be received with or without surrounding tunica vaginalis, and with or without attached spermatic cord (**104, 105**). If present, the tunica vaginalis should be opened, noting the presence of any hydrocele, so that the external surface of the testis can be examined.

Measurements are then made of the testis, epididymis and cord. Clinically, testes are measured by comparison with a set of graded ovoids; the size is recorded in millilitres, the normal range being 15-25 ml. In the laboratory, testes are usually measured in centimetres, but to allow clinical correlation the volume can easily be found by immersing the testis in water in a measuring cylinder and recording the volume displaced.

Formalin diffuses slowly through the fibrous tunica albuginea immediately surrounding the testis, and the specimen should be bisected longitudinally from the anteromedial aspect through to the epididymis (**104, 105, 106**). This is best done by the pathologist after the fresh specimen has been measured, preferably as soon as possible after its arrival in the laboratory. The specimen can then be fixed without delay. Bisection can cause distortion because of contraction of the tunica and eversion of the testicular tubules or tumour, but in practice this is usually preferable to inadequate fixation.

Dense white scar tissue is easily recognizable in an otherwise normal sandy-brown, finely granular testis (**104**). Haemorrhagic areas in particular should be carefully sampled. In tumours, these may simply represent degeneration but might in some cases contain trophoblastic teratoma.

Blocks should be taken from testicular neoplasms as shown in **106b**. Several blocks should be taken from the tumour and adjacent uninvolved testis, the tunica albuginea, the tunica vaginalis and the epididymis. Blocks should also be taken from the excision line of the spermatic cord, from its centre, and from the lower end adjacent to the upper pole of the testis. For orchiec-tomies performed for non-neoplastic disease, two or three blocks should be taken from the testis, especially from focal lesions or variegated areas, and from the epididymis, tunica vaginalis and spermatic cord if present.

Testis: Macroscopical report	
Type of specimen	Unilateral orchiectomy, orchiectomy with spermatic cord
Measurements	Overall dimensions of entire specimen Size and weight of testis and epididymis and/or volume of the testis Length and diameter of spermatic cord
Description	
External appearance	Dilated veins, loss of normal shiny appearance (which might indicate microscopic involvement by tumour), obvious tumour spread through the tunica
Cut surface	Colour and uniformity (diffuse pink and white tissue, variegated grey, red and white areas, clear mucinous areas); consistency (soft, rubbery, hard, friable); contour (well-circumscribed, ill-defined); tissues involved by tumour (tunica albuginea, tunica vaginalis, epididymis, scrotum, spermatic cord); testis away from the lesion, if any remains
Rest of specimen	Surrounding tunica vaginalis, epididymis, presence of hydrocele

Example 105-106

An orchiectomy specimen consisting of a testis measuring 3.8 × 4.5 × 7 cm with attached tunica vaginalis, epididymis and 5.5 cm of spermatic cord. The tunica vaginalis appears congested, but has a normal shiny appearance. The cut surface of the testis shows a well-defined tumour measuring 3.7 × 4 × 6.8 cm composed of white tissue in which there are small, irregular red areas compatible with recent haemorrhage. No residual normal testis is apparent. The tumour extends into but not through the tunica albuginea and invades the inferior pole of the epididymis. The spermatic cord shows no macroscopical abnormality; there is no evidence of tumour spread on cross sections from the lower, middle or upper ends.

Blocks

- A centre of tumour × 2
- B tumour and area of epididymis × 2
- C tumour and tunicas × 2
- D tumour and uninvolved testis × 1
- E resection end of cord × 1
- F middle of cord × 1
- G lower end of cord × 1

Epididymis and vas

The epididymis may be biopsied for inflammation or neoplasia. The tissue received will be small and difficult to orientate, and the whole specimen should be embedded. Epididymal cysts and adenomatoid tumours provide larger specimens in which parallel cuts should be made through the tissue, and blocks taken especially from cyst walls, areas of solid tissue and foci of haemorrhage. If the lesion is found as part of an orchiectomy specimen (**107**), it should be measured, described and treated as for testicular neoplasms.

Vasa deferentia in cases of sterilization should be received in separate pots with the site of origin specified. After measuring, a short cylinder should be removed from the centre of the specimen. With small lengths of vas, half of the specimen should be taken. Wherever possible, at least a short length of vas is retained unprocessed, so that a report will still be possible if there is a failure in the tissue processing.

Epididymis and vas: Macroscopical report	
Type of specimen	Tissue fragment, nodule, cord of tissue, thin-walled cyst
Measurements	Maximum dimensions or diameter
Description	Colour Consistency (firm, hard, soft, cystic) Cyst contents (clear thin fluid, blood-stained fluid)

104

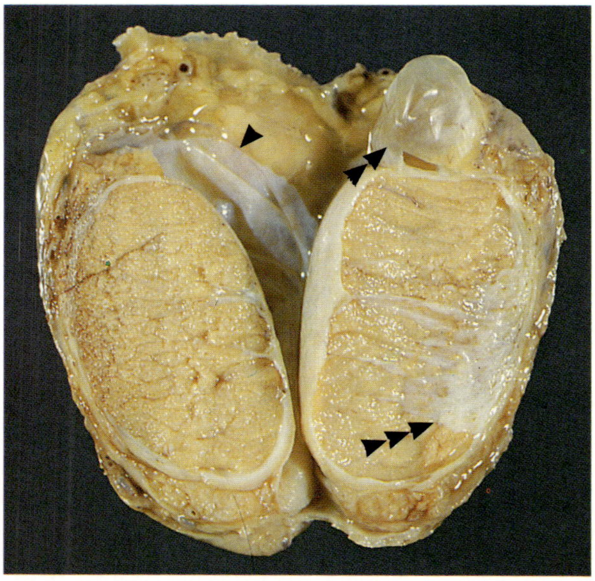

104 A testis with surrounding tunica vaginalis (▶) removed for palliative treatment of prostatic carcinoma. The specimen has been bisected and shows a small epididymal cyst at the upper pole (▶▶) and focal scarring of the testis posteriorly (▶▶▶).

105 The outer aspect of an enlarged testis with attached spermatic cord. The tunica vaginalis is smooth and shiny.

106a On sectioning 105, the normal testicular tissue has been completely replaced by a tumour which has the typical solid white appearance of a seminoma.

105

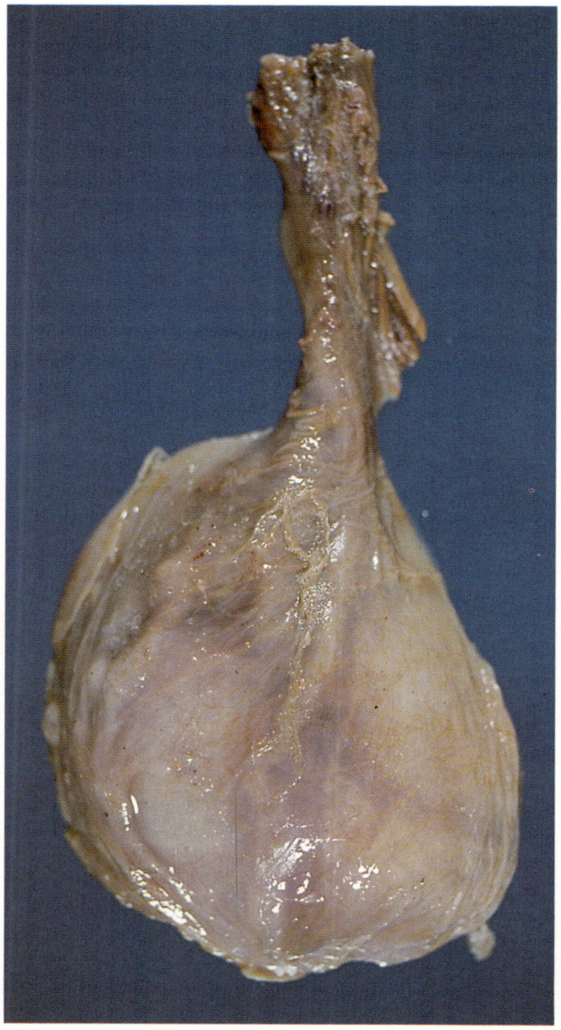

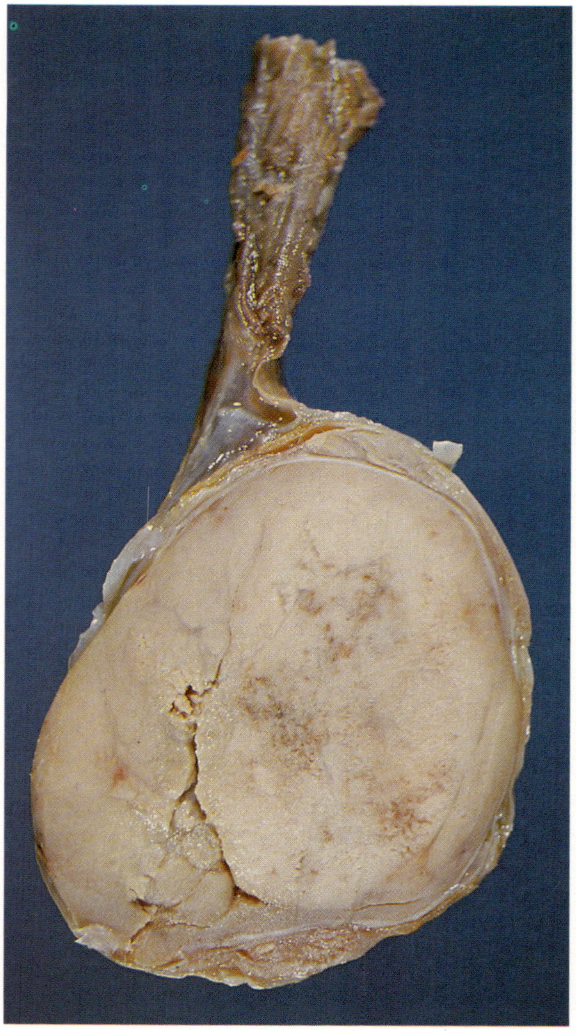

106a

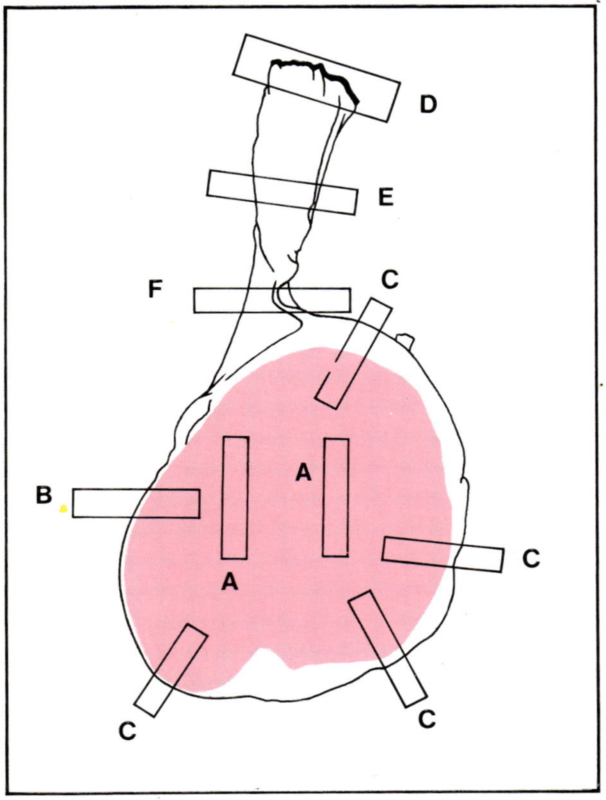

106b Blocks taken from an orchiectomy specimen with suspected or proven neoplasia: centre of tumour (**A**); tumour and area of epididymus (**B**); tumour and tunicas (**C**); excision end of cord (**D**); middle of cord (**E**); lower end of cord (**F**). If any normal testis remains, a block is also taken from this.

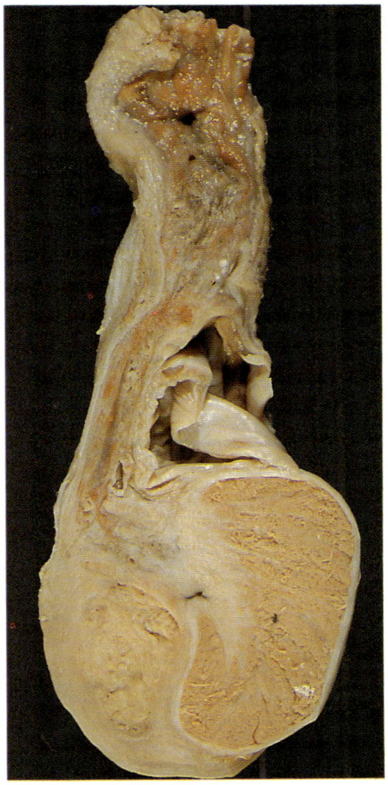

107 An orchiectomy specimen showing tuberculous epididymitis. Caseous material has replaced much of the body of the epididymis. This testis was removed because the lesion was thought to be a testicular neoplasm.

Prostate

Small specimens

Prostatic biopsies and resections are performed for inflammation, hyperplasia and carcinoma. The commonest prostatic biopsies are transurethral curettings obtained through a resectoscope, mainly from the middle, lateral and anterior lobes of the gland (**108**). The amount received can range from a few grams to over 60 g, and will depend on whether the purpose of resection was to provide tissue for histological diagnosis of prostatic disease, to relieve obstructive symptoms, or both.

It is possible to assess the size of a patient's prostate ultrasonically, and clinicians may find it useful for clinicopathological correlation to have the volume removed recorded accurately. Aggregated curettings may be measured roughly with a ruler, but a better method is to measure volume by displacement of water in a measuring cylinder. The weight of the tissue fragments is also recorded. It does not indicate the percentage of the prostate excised, as the weight of the whole gland cannot be established, but it may be useful to indicate to the surgeon whether the excision was modest, average or extensive.

The selection of fragments should not be random. Those that are focally or diffusely yellow should be selected, as they are more likely to be infiltrated by adenocarcinoma (**108**). Malignant prostatic tissue tends to be yellower than benign tissue because the carcinoma cells contain more cytoplasmic

Prostate: Macroscopical report	
Type of specimen	Transurethral resection, retropubic prostatectomy, prostatectomy with cystectomy
Measurements	Weight of tissue Range of sizes of nodules
Description	
Outer surface	Contour (nodular, irregular); presence of and appearance of prostatic urethra
Cut surface	Colour (white, milky, yellow, focal lesions); uniformity (nodular, focally diffuse)

lipid than normal and are present in greater numbers.

The number of blocks taken from prostatic curettings varies widely. One cassette may be taken for every 5 or 10 g of the specimen, but it has been found that five cassettes of prostatic curettings will reveal virtually all the possible pathology present, irrespective of the total weight of tissue resected.

Some surgeons practise differential curettage. The fragments from the different parts of the gland should be weighed and put into separately labelled cassettes.

Needle biopsy, obtained with a Tru-cut or similar biopsy needle through the perineum or anterior rectal wall, may be used in the diagnosis of malignancy. The core of tissue is measured and the whole specimen processed, preferably laid flat on a piece of card or wrapped in tissue paper to facilitate embedding in one plane. Because of the paucity of the sample, step or serial sections should be requested.

The macroscopical report can be limited to, for example, 'prostatic curettings, together measuring . . . and weighing . . . . Two thirds embedded in five cassettes', or 'a needle core of pale tissue measuring . . . in length. All embedded'.

Large specimens

Retropubic prostatectomy and other incisional prostate operations provide large amounts of tissue, often 100 g or more (**109**). The specimen should be measured, weighed and sectioned every 5 mm at right angles to the prostatic urethra, if this can be identified. One block at least should include the mucosal surface of the urethra, and the subcapsular area should be extensively sampled to look for malignant disease. Where the orientation of the specimen is not evident, parallel cuts are made at similar intervals through any axis. Blocks should be taken especially of homogeneous pale pink or yellow areas of tissue.

Example 109-110
The specimen consists of two rounded masses of rubbery tissue, both of which are approximately spherical and measure 2.5 cm in diameter. Together they weigh 34 g. No urethra is identified. The cut surface shows multiple nodules of white tissue ranging from 0.4-0.9 cm in diameter in which there are numerous tiny cystic spaces containing milky white fluid.

Blocks × 4

108 A transurethral resection of the prostate. The yellow areas (▶) were found histologically to be adenocarcinoma. The rest of the specimen showed benign hyperplasia.

108

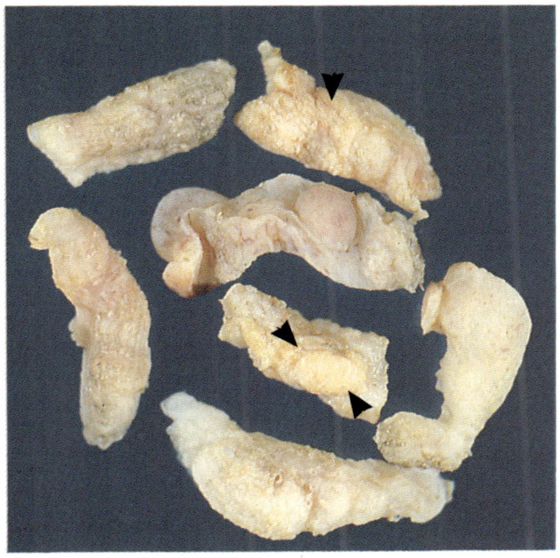

109 A retropubic prostatectomy specimen comprising two rounded multinodular masses of rubbery tissue.

109

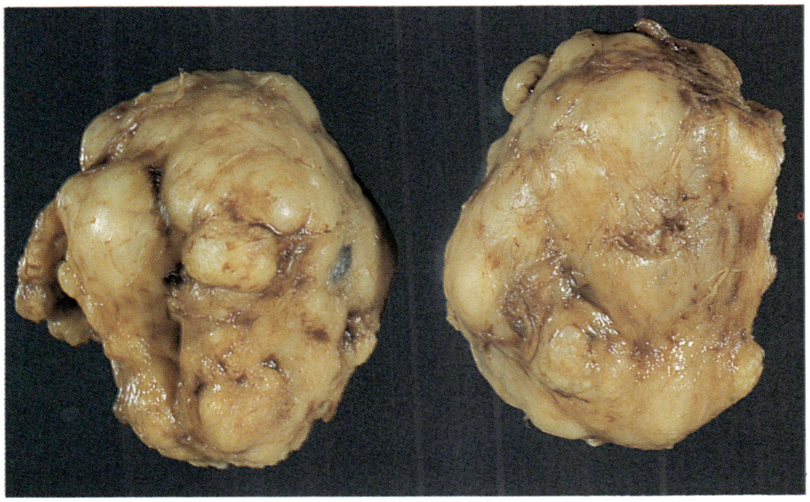

110 A section of 109 revealing a white and lobulated cut surface with numerous tiny cystic spaces. Histologically the prostate was found to show benign nodular hyperplasia.

110

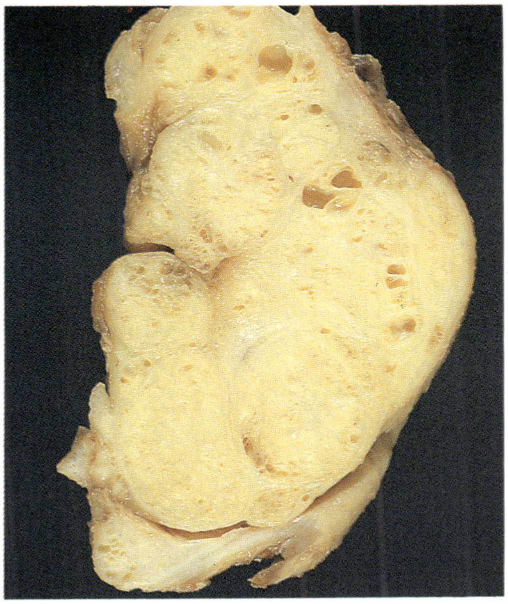

Penis and scrotum

Small specimens

Biopsies from the skin of the penis and scrotum for inflammatory conditions, viral warts or malignant neoplasms should be treated as for skin biopsies (p 97).

Sheets of foreskin removed at circumcision are seldom diseased in infants and children, but in adults they may require pathological examination to investigate inflammatory changes, lichen sclerosus (balanitis xerotica obliterans) and Bowen's disease. Description of a sheet of foreskin is normally short (for example 'A sheet of pale rugose skin measuring . . . '). The appearances and extent of any pathological changes should be recorded, and blocks taken transversely across the specimen.

The penile urethra may be removed as part of the treatment of multifocal urothelial malignancy, and should be treated as described on p 88.

Penile amputation

Amputations of the penis may be performed for carcinoma and trauma, for 'sex-change' procedures and, very rarely, for inflammatory conditions that have resulted in severe distortion and pain.

Dissection of specimen

After fixation, a penile amputation specimen should be measured and examined. Carcinoma of the penis most commonly affects the glans and coronal sulcus as a white, exophytic mass which infiltrates into the corpora cavernosa and may spread through them (**111**, **112**). It may be impossible macroscopically to determine the proximal extent of the tumour. A rare type of squamous cell carcinoma of the penis is verrucous carcinoma (carcinoma cuniculatum and giant condyloma of Buschke-Löwenstein are considered to be the same condition). This presents as a very slow-growing warty growth which may appear superficially to be a viral condyloma but which infiltrates into the underlying corpora with blunt, rounded projections.

The description of a penis or penile tissues removed because of trauma should record the type of injury (burns, crush injury, traction, 'degloving' or removal of the skin from the shaft) as well as the macroscopical features, and a photographic record should be made if possible.

Before dissection, blocks should be taken from the skin, corpora and urethra at the excision end (**112b**), in order to look for involvement by tumour or to assess the viability of injured tissues. Beginning at the external meatus, the urethra is opened through the ventral aspect where it runs

Penis: Macroscopical report	
Type of specimen	Foreskin, penile amputation, sheet of rugose skin
Measurements	Length, width and thickness of foreskin Length of amputation specimen from external meatus to excision line, diameter of shaft
Description	
Tumour	Size; site; distance from excision margin; colour; growth pattern (fungating, papillary, warty, ulcerated); consistency (friable, soft, rubbery); contour (well-defined, indistinct, 'pushing' margins) Adjacent tissues (infiltration, induration or congestion of foreskin, frenulum, glans, meatus, urethra, corpora cavernosa, corpus spongiosum)
Trauma	Skin (ulceration, contusions, burns, lacerations, extent of loss of, degloving); deep tissues (haemorrhage, induration); urethra (congested, intraluminal haemorrhage)

closest to the overlying skin. A long-bladed knife can then be inserted into this cut, and the penis bisected longitudinally (**111, 112a**). In most cases this will demonstrate the pathology satisfactorily, and if necessary further cuts can be made through the halves of the specimen at right angles to the shaft. The extent of tumour spread or severity of injury to the different structures and compartments (foreskin, frenulum, glans, meatus, corpora cavernosa, urethra and corpus spongiosum) should be assessed.

Blocks are taken from the tumour, the adjacent urethra and any other lesions away from the tumour (**112b**). Biopsies or excisions of large condylomatous lesions should be extensively sampled to assess the depth and nature of the extension into the adjacent tissues.

111 A penile amputation specimen (external surface). The glans penis and distal shaft are expanded by an exophytic tumour mass showing focal surface ulceration.

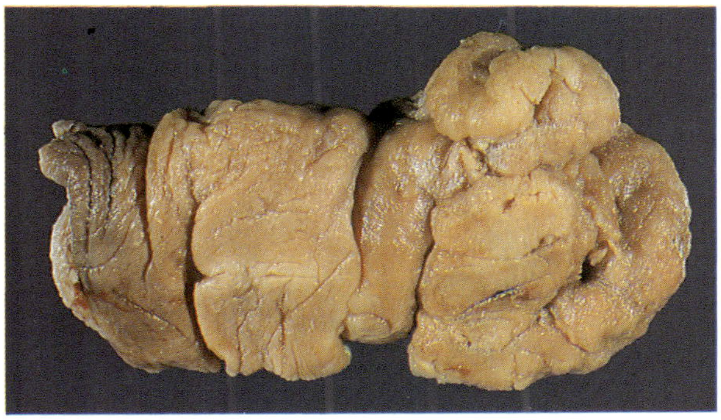

111

112a A section of the tumour in 111 showing a dense white cut surface. The tumour has completely replaced the normal tissues of the distal third of the organ with partial occlusion of the penile urethra (▶).

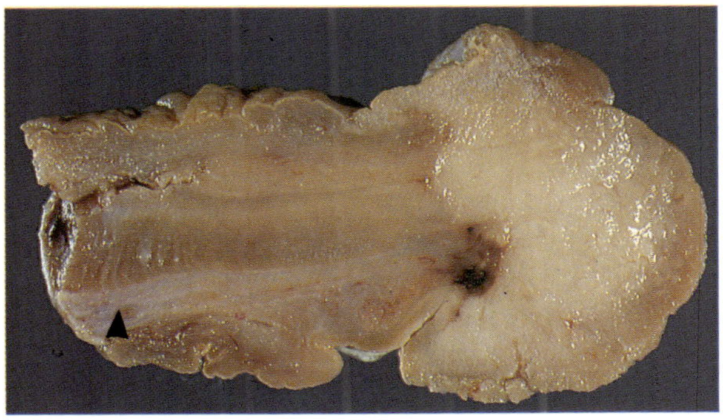

112a

112b Blocks taken from a penile amputation specimen: dorsal penile excision margin (**A**); ventral penile and urethral excision margins (**B**); tumour (**C**); tumour and adjacent urethra (**D**); middle third of specimen (**E**); proximal third of specimen (**F**).

112b

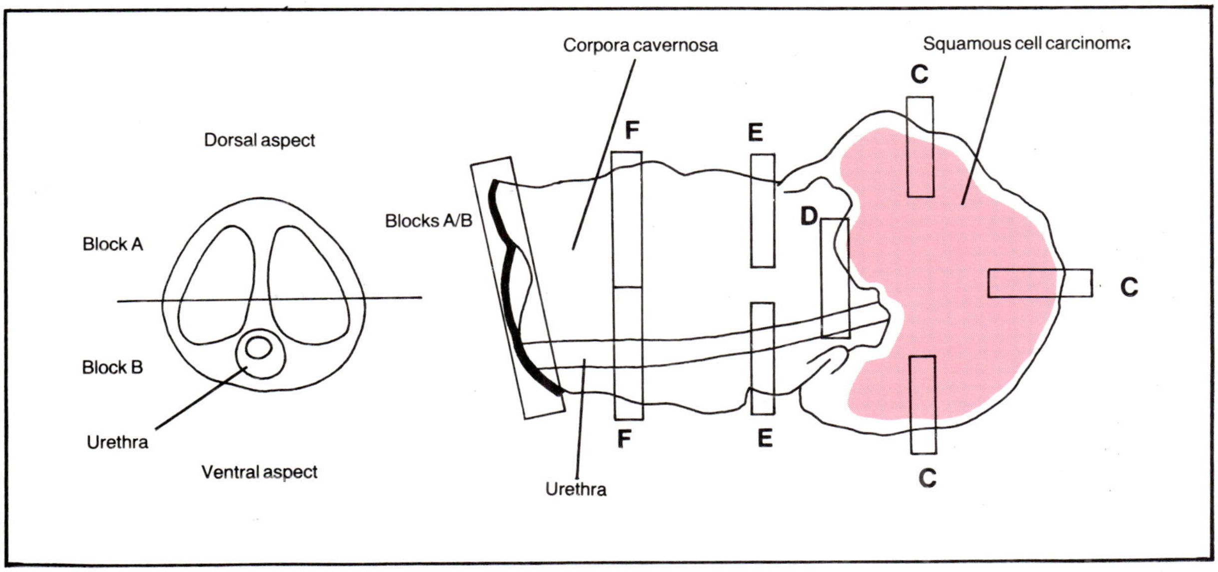

CHAPTER 6
URINARY TRACT

Kidney

Small specimens

Needle biopsy of the kidney, used for the investigation of parenchymal renal disease and renal transplant rejection, is the only small specimen taken with any frequency. The biopsy should be received fresh and examined as soon as possible, so that a further biopsy may be taken if necessary. Glomeruli can be seen under the dissecting microscope as tiny red dots or smudges (**113**). Unhealthy glomeruli contain fewer red cells and may be difficult to identify. The medulla appears as white tissue with pink streaks.

The treatment of the tissue will depend on its size and the presence or absence of obvious glomeruli on examination under the dissecting microscope, but most of all it will depend on the suspected clinical diagnosis. Diagnosis of many renal diseases requires immunofluorescence and electron microscopical examination as well as light microscopy, and if necessary, tissue for freezing and glutaraldehyde fixation is taken at this stage. When enough tissue is available, two or three 1 mm lengths should be taken from the cortex for electron microscope examination, the same number frozen for immunofluorescence, and the rest of the tissue processed, without further cutting, into paraffin wax or resin. The description is limited to, for example, 'A core of pink and white tissue measuring . . . in which glomerular tufts can be identified under the dissecting microscope'.

Large specimens

A kidney may be removed for tumour (usually carcinoma), intractable unilateral obstruction and/or inflammation in which the renal parenchyma is largely destroyed, and for the treatment of some forms of hypertension. Partial nephrectomy specimens are unusual except in cases where the patient has had a previous contralateral nephrectomy.

Dissection of specimen
The approach to dissection will depend upon the reason for nephrectomy.

Nephrectomy for carcinoma
Nephrectomy specimens for carcinoma are usually received with surrounding adipose tissue (**114**). The entire specimen should be measured, then, leaving the perinephric fat *in situ*, it should be sliced coronally from the lateral border so that the cut bisects the kidney and opens the renal pelvis (**115a**). The halves may be separated or the medial part left intact to form a 'hinge' (**115a, 116, 117**). This approach will display the pathology present in almost all cases. Further fixation is usually necessary at this stage, and a photographic record is recommended, especially if focal lesions are apparent.

When fully fixed, the excision margins of the main renal vessels and the ureter should be taken before the specimen is dissected further, so that translocation of tumour into these structures is avoided as far as possible. A search should be made for lymph nodes in the perinephric fat around the renal hilum (it is unusual for nodes to be found elsewhere in the specimen). The adrenal gland should also be sought in the perinephric fat, then dissected free, weighed, measured and examined for tumour involvement.

The next step is to establish the relation between the tumour and the overlying capsule and adipose tissue. At this stage the adipose tissue may be removed from the renal capsule (which is left attached to the kidney) and extrarenal spread of tumour should be noted (**116**). This is especially important for renal parenchymal cell carcinoma, but transitional cell carcinoma of the renal pelvis occasionally

Nephrectomy: Macroscopical report	
Type of specimen	Partial nephrectomy, total nephrectomy with perinephric adipose tissue
Measurements	Thickness of perinephric adipose tissue if present Size and weight of the kidney Length of ureter
Description	
Focal lesions if present	Size; site (upper pole, centre, pelvis, etc.); contour (rounded, papillary, irregular); colour (renal parenchymal cell carcinoma is often variegated); consistency (caseous, mucoid, rubbery) Extent of involvement of adjacent kidney, capsule, perinephric adipose tissue, calyces and pelvis, blood vessels, around hilum
Rest of kidney	*Renal capsule* Appearance (easily removed, focally adherent, scarred, densely fibrosed); relation with surrounding adipose tissue *Surface* Fetal lobulations, smooth, finely granular, congested, coarsely scarred, abscess formation *Cortex* Thickness; colour; demarcation from medulla *Medulla* Colour; appearance of pyramids (blunted, calcified, distorted, congested) *Pelvicalyceal system* Dilated, distorted, congested, stenosis; presence of calculi, pus *Ureter* Dilated above a lesion, involved by tumour from outside the ureter, inflamed *Vascular pedicle* Atheroma, fibromuscular stenosis *Lymph nodes* Hilar lymph nodes (number, appearance)
Adrenal gland	Size; weight; appearance (atrophic, nodular, involved by tumour)

spreads into the adjacent tissues. The ureter and vessels are then opened and examined for involvement by tumour.

The size and weight of the kidney, the length of the attached ureter and the thicknesses of the non-neoplastic cortex should be recorded.

Blocks are taken from the tumour and adjacent parenchyma, the overlying capsule and adipose tissue, the uninvolved cortex and medulla, the pelvis and ureter, the vascular and ureteric excision margins, and the hilar lymph nodes (**115b**).

Nephrectomy for non-neoplastic disease

The method for handling the specimen is similar to that described above for carcinoma, except that on receipt the capsule is stripped away from the surface of the kidney with the perinephric fat (**118, 119**). This can be done before the kidney is bisected. Excision margins and hilar lymph nodes are not usually important in these cases. The sites and appearance of any calculi should be recorded. Chemical analysis is seldom of diagnostic value but X-ray energy dispersive spectroscopy on tissue sections or fragments of calculus may occasionally reveal unexpected components such as silica. The condition of the renal papillae and pelvic mucosa should be examined, and the presence of hydronephrosis, strictures or distortion of the pelvicalyceal system should be noted.

Example 114-115

The specimen consists of a kidney measuring 5 × 6.6 × 8 cm and weighing 90 g, surrounded by a layer of adipose tissue up to 4 cm thick. A 16 cm length of ureter is attached.

There is a large tumour mass arising in the area of the lower and middle calyces which infiltrates the adjacent parenchyma and extends into the pelvis and down the first 3 cm of the ureter. The tumour measures 5.1 × 3 × 2.2 cm and is composed of friable brown tissue in which there are several areas of haemorrhage. There is no evidence of invasion of the renal capsule or the perinephric fat. Adjacent to the tumour the cortex is thinned, and measures 0.4 cm. Elsewhere, the corticomedullary junction is indistinct. The pelvicalyceal system away from the tumour is dilated. The distal ureter measures 0.5 cm in diameter and does not appear to be involved by tumour. The renal vessels at the hilum show no evidence of tumour invasion. Three small hilar lymph nodes are found. No adrenal gland is present in the perinephric fat.

Blocks

- A hilar vessels × 1
- B hilar lymph nodes × 3
- C ureteric excision line × 1
- D tumour and calyceal system × 2
- E tumour and adjacent parenchyma × 1
- F tumour and overlying renal capsule × 3
- G focal yellow lesion × 1
- H, J uninvolved upper and lower pole of renal parenchyma × 2
- K proximal ureter × 1

113 A needle biopsy of the kidney. The glomeruli can be seen as tiny red dots (▶) and the medulla as white tissue with pink streaks. In kidneys with glomerular disease, in which the blood supply to the glomeruli is decreased, glomeruli may be very difficult to identify.

113

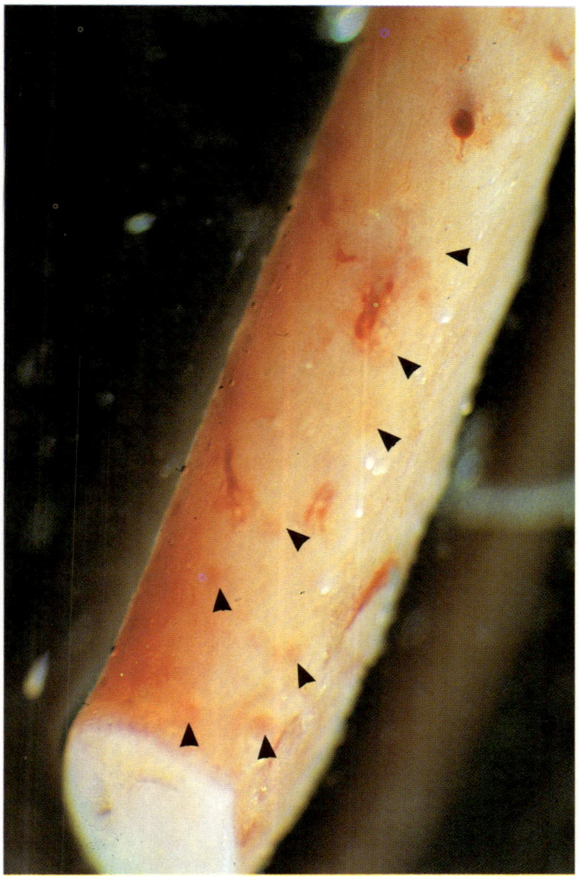

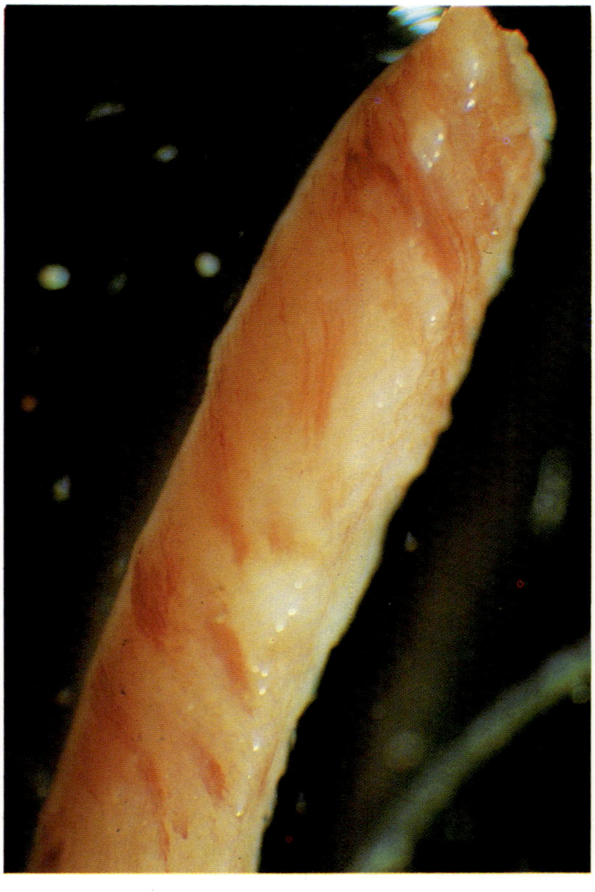

114 A total nephrectomy specimen, outer aspect. The perinephric adipose tissue is intact. The ureter protrudes from its lower pole. Ligatures around the renal hilar vessels can be seen in the centre of the figure (▶).

114

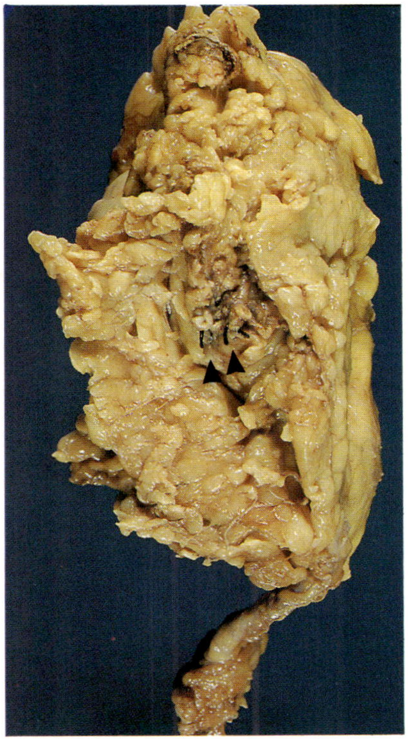

115a Specimen 114 bisected to reveal a tumour mass within the renal pelvis.

115a

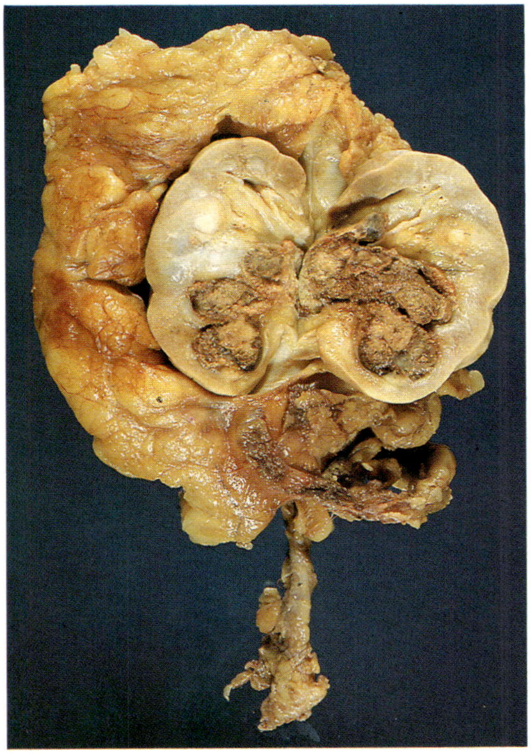

115b

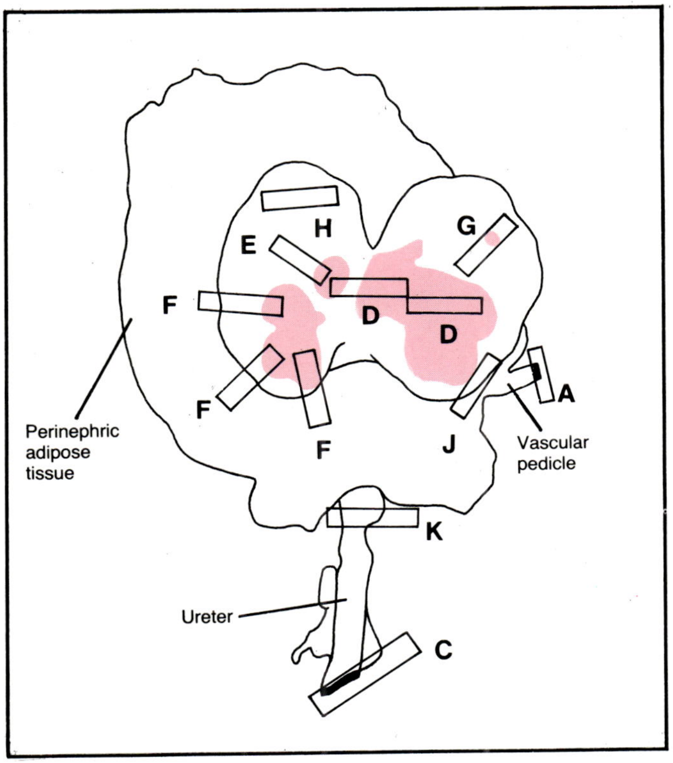

115b Blocks taken from a nephrectomy specimen containing a tumour: hilar vessels (**A**); hilar lymph nodes (**B**—not shown); ureteric excision margin (**C**); tumour (**D**); tumour and adjacent parenchyma (**E**); tumour and overlying renal capsule (**F**—especially important with renal cell carcinomas); any other focal lesion (**G**); uninvolved upper and lower pole renal parenchyma (**H** and **J**); proximal ureter (**K**).

116

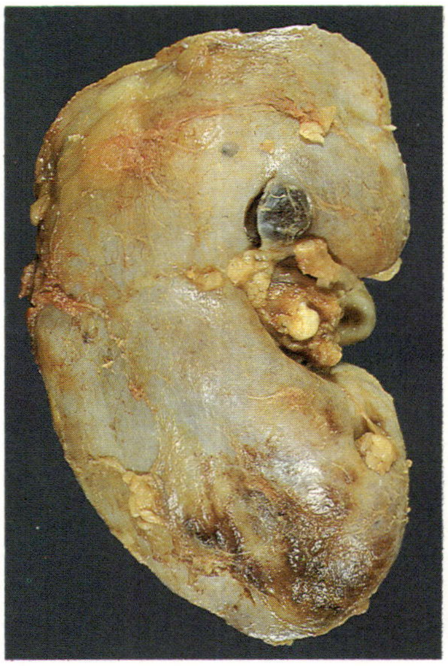

117

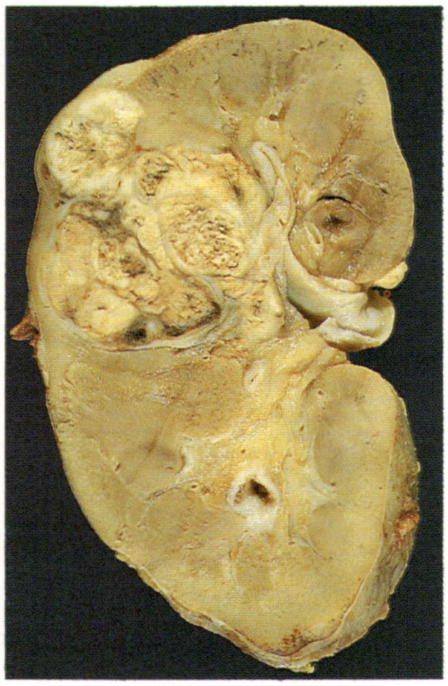

116 Nephrectomy performed for renal parenchymal cell carcinoma. After blocks are taken from the vascular and ureteric excision margins, and a search made for hilar lymph nodes, the perinephric fat is dissected away leaving the renal capsule intact and the kidney bisected. No evidence of involvement of the perinephric fat was found in this specimen.

117 The cut surface of 116 showing a tumour with a nodular, yellow, variegated cut surface typical of renal parenchymal cell carcinoma.

118

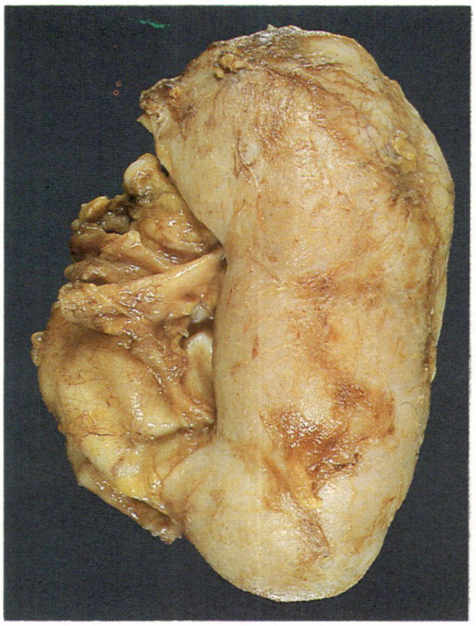

119

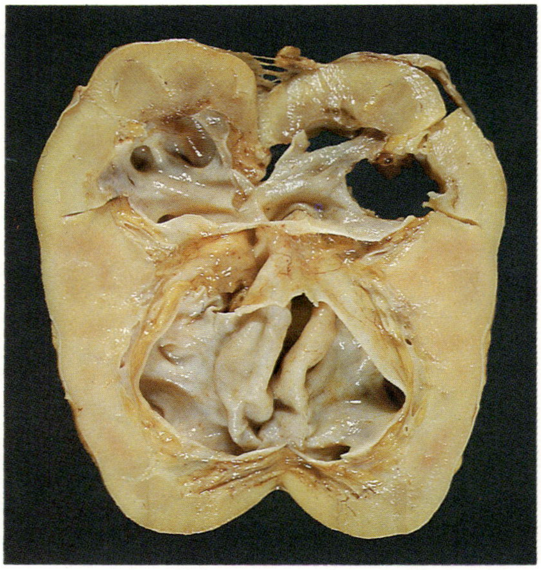

118 A hydronephrotic kidney with severely dilated renal pelvis. When a kidney is removed because of intractable inflammation or other non-neoplastic disease, the perinephric fat can be removed before the kidney is incised.

119 The cut surface of 118 showing that the dilatation involves the calyceal system. The cortex and medulla are thinner than normal. There is little macroscopical evidence of pyelitis or pyelonephritis.

Ureter

Lengths of ureter are excised with nephrectomy and cystectomy specimens, but short lengths of ureter may sometimes be removed for benign stricture, or very rarely for neoplasia where the patient has a solitary kidney. The length and diameter (or average and maximum diameters if there is focal dilatation) of the cord of tissue are measured. Transverse sections of the excision margins are blocked. If there is a stricture, transverse cuts are made along the length of the specimen and blocks taken of the pre-stenotic, stenotic and post-stenotic areas. If a carcinoma is suspected, the ureter is opened longitudinally and blocks taken of the tumour and the underlying wall, and of the wall away from the lesion. The description of the specimen should be similar to that for ureters attached to cystectomy specimens below.

Bladder

Small specimens

Cystoscopic biopsies are commonly taken to investigate inflammatory conditions and neoplasia. The quantity of tissue can vary from a single tiny biopsy to large numbers of fragments of papillary tumour. Orientation is usually impossible, and all of the fragments are embedded unless a very large quantity is received. If a transitional cell carcinoma has been biopsied, selection of fragments for blocks should not be random. Firm, solid tissue is more likely to contain invasive tumour and bladder muscularis, allowing a better assessment of the depth of the tumour spread than papillary fragments.

In most cases the macroscopical report is limited to, for example, 'A fragment of pink tissue measuring . . . ' or 'Numerous fronded fragments of pink and brown tissue 2 × 2 × 1 cm in aggregate volume. All embedded'.

Large specimens

Cystectomy or partial cystectomy may be performed for neoplasms not controlled by conservative measures, and for intractable inflammation or radiation damage with pain, distortion and loss of function. Specimens may consist of the fundus of the bladder, parts of the anterior or posterior walls or the entire bladder. In cystectomy for malignancy, the prostate and urethra are often removed, and other pelvic organs may also be excised (**120, 121, 122, 123**).

Initial dissection

Sheets of bladder wall should be pinned out flat and left to fix further. There are several ways of handling total cystectomy specimens. They should first be orientated, using the peritoneal reflections over the anterior and posterior surfaces (**120, 121, 122, 124, 125**) and the insertion of the ureters as guides. The position of the seminal vesicles (**121**) or the uterus (**122**), if present, will also be useful.

If the bladder has been incised anteriorly or posteriorly before receipt in the laboratory, it is usually best to continue the incisions as necessary to allow the specimen to be pinned out flat (**124, 126, 127, 128a**). If the specimen is intact or has been cut through the lateral aspect, it should be bisected coronally and left to fix further (**123**). An alternative method with intact specimens is to distend the lumen with formalin, either via the urethra, with a Foley catheter, or by injection directly through the wall. Expansion may be difficult if there has been previous radiotherapy to the bladder and in any case great care should be taken when injecting formalin. The specimen is then left immersed in formalin to fix. After fixation the bladder is divided into anterior and posterior halves (bisection sagittally will distort the relations of the trigone, ureteric orifices and bladder neck).

Dissection of specimen

The specimen should be photographed if possible and if there is a doubt about the excision margins, these should be marked with India ink. With sheets of bladder wall, blocks should be taken radially to show the nearest extensions of the tumour to the lateral excision margins. Parallel cuts are then made through the tumour to reveal the depth of invasion towards the deep excision line, and several blocks should be taken.

With total cystectomy specimens, it is advisable first to identify the ureters, urethra, seminal vesicles and other structures present. Complete transverse sections are taken from the excision margins of the ureters and urethra, and from the prostatic excision line if the tumour appears to involve the trigone and prostatic urethra. The urethra is opened along its dorsal aspect and transverse blocks are taken of any lesions present. Parallel transverse cuts are made through the ureters starting extravesically, to investigate involvement by tumour. Opening longitudinally with fine scissors is an alternative method, but it can be difficult to open the intravesical portion of the ureters without distorting the specimen.

A series of close parallel cuts is then made through the tumour to assess the depth of invasion and infiltration of surrounding structures, and blocks are taken from these slices (**128b**).

Cystectomy: Macroscopical report	
Type of specimen	Partial cystectomy, total cystectomy with excision of seminal vesicles, prostate, lower ureters and urethra and surrounding adipose tissue Other structures present
Measurements	Dimensions of sheets of bladder wall, or overall size of total cystectomy specimen as maximum dimensions Sizes of the bladder, prostate Lengths of ureters, urethra
Description	
Focal lesions	Type (tumour, plaque, ulcer, scar); site (anterior wall and trigone, around left ureteric orifice, etc.); size and number; colour; contour (papillary, solid invasive, flat diffuse, rolled edges); consistency (necrotic, friable, firm); extent of spread, and tissues involved
Rest of specimen	
Bladder wall	Discoloration of mucosa; abnormal consistency (boggy, firm); presence of thickening and trabeculation
Serosa	Adhesions, distortion, fibrinous exudate
Ureters	Length, diameter at different sites (dilatation above a stricture, above the ureteric orifices because of involvement by carcinoma); appearance of mucosa and wall
Other tissues	Prostate, seminal vesicles, urethra, uterus, etc. (macroscopically normal, hyperplasia, congestion)

Example 124-126

A radical cystectomy specimen consisting of the bladder, prostate, seminal vesicles, lower ureters and surrounding connective tissue. The bladder measures 15 × 9 × 8 cm. The posterior wall and trigone are replaced by a fungating grey and brown tumour mass measuring 6 × 5 cm, and 3 cm in thickness. The cut surface suggests that the tumour is confined to the lamina propria and inner layers of the muscularis. Both ureteric orifices are surrounded by tumour but there is no ureteric dilatation.. Away from the tumour, the bladder mucosa has numerous petechial haemorrhages. The ureters each measure 4.5 cm long and 0.8 cm in diameter. The prostate shows nodular enlargement. The seminal vesicles appear normal. Two small lymph nodes are identified in the periurethral fat.

Blocks

A	excision margin of left ureter × 1
B	excision margin of right ureter × 1
C	excision margin of prostatic urethra and prostate × 3
D	posterior wall and trigone of bladder with tumour × 1
E	left lateral wall of bladder × 1
F	right lateral wall of bladder × 1
G	anterior wall of bladder × 1
H	left seminal vesicles × 1
J	right seminal vesicles × 1
K	lymph node in right perivesical fat × 1
L	lymph node in left perivesical fat × 1

120

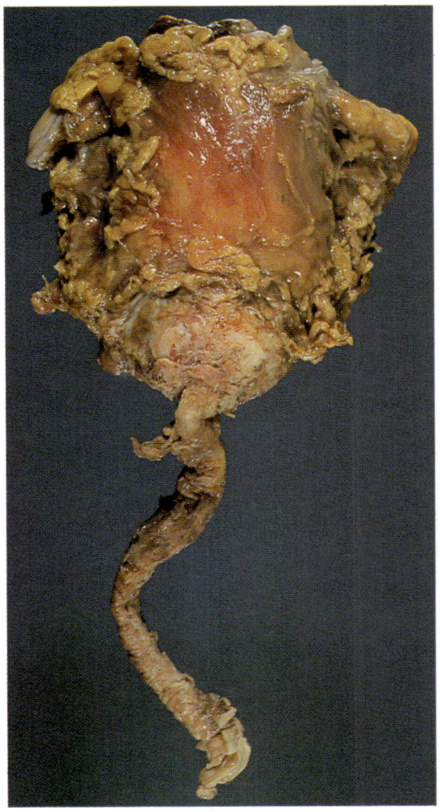

121

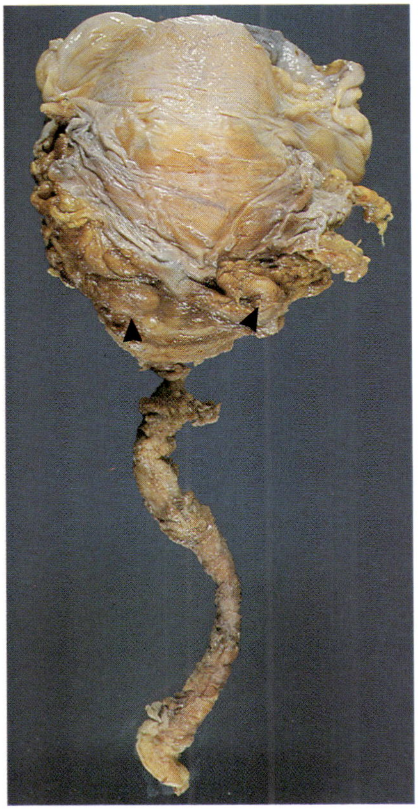

120 The anterior aspect of a cystectomy and urethrectomy specimen. The peritoneum covers the dome of the bladder and upper anterior wall; the lower part is covered by adipose tissue. The urethra has been excised as far as the external penile meatus.

121 The same specimen as 120. On the posterior aspect the peritoneal reflection descends further and the seminal vesicles (▶) are apparent.

122

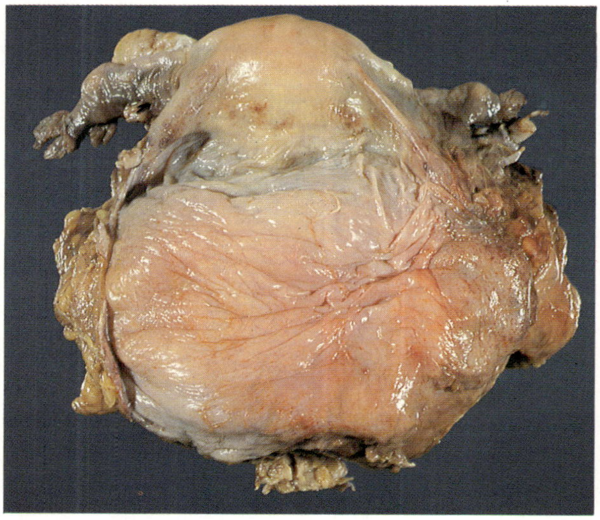

122 A combined cystectomy/hysterectomy specimen (anterior surface).

123

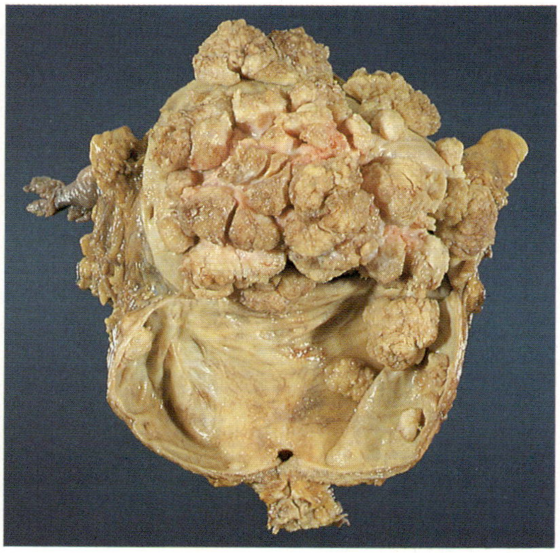

123 The bladder in 122 opened in the coronal plane through the urethra, leaving the anterior and posterior halves attached at the dome. A large fungating tumour is present on the anterior wall.

124

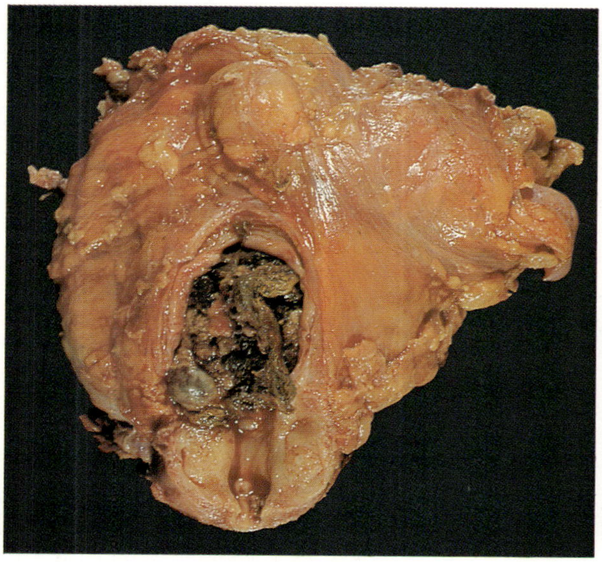

124 The anterior surface of a cystectomy specimen from a male patient. The specimen has been partly opened prior to receipt.

125

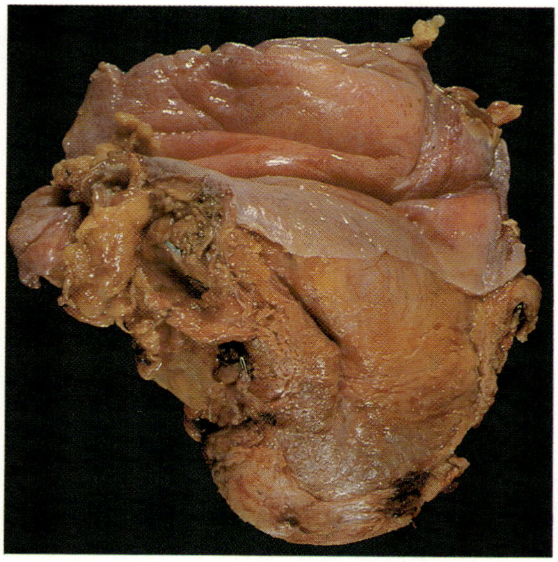

125 The posterior surface of the bladder shown in 124. The peritoneum has retracted since the specimen was excised, but it is still lower over the posterior aspect than over the anterior.

126 The cut in the anterior wall of 124 has been extended superiorly and laterally in a T-shape to allow the specimen to be pinned out. A large necrotic tumour is attached to the inferior two thirds of the posterior wall.

126

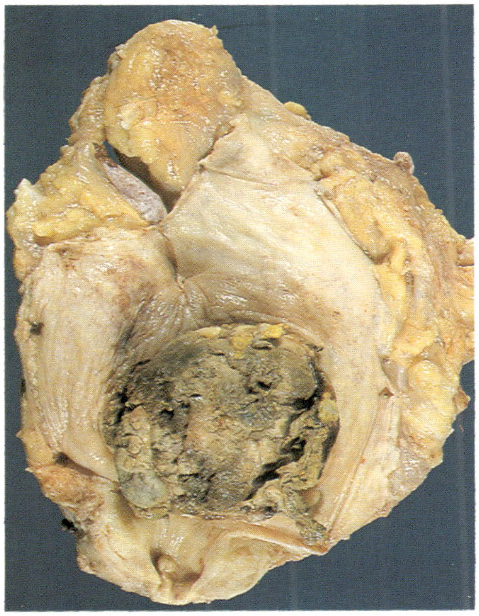

127 The anterior surface of a cystectomy specimen from a male patient. A small incision was made in the prostatic urethra and the inferior part of the bladder in the operating theatre.

128a The anterior incision in the bladder in 127 has been extended superiorly and laterally in a T-shape and the specimen pinned out. The bladder wall is severely thickened and a papillary tumour occupies most of the mucosal surface. The prostate is also moderately enlarged.

127

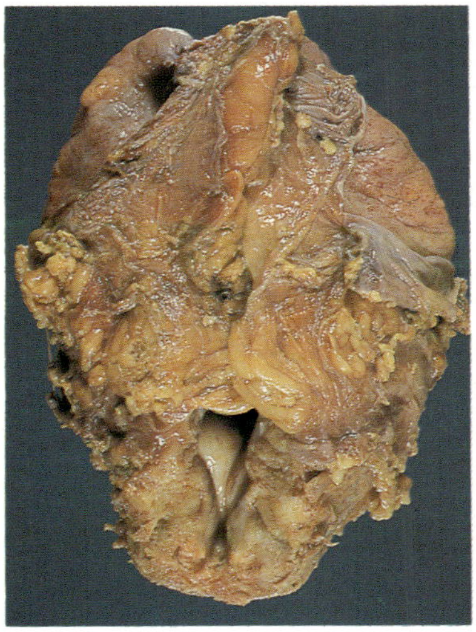

128a

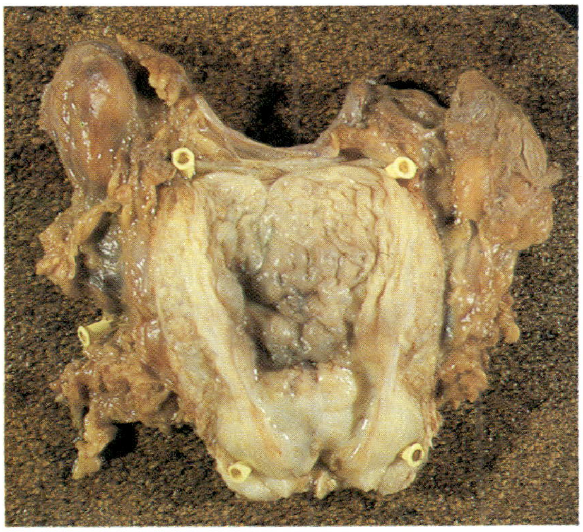

128b Blocks taken from a cystectomy specimen: full thickness blocks of anterior, right lateral, posterior, left lateral and superior bladder wall and tumour (**A, B, C, D, E**); excision margin of prostate and prostatic urethra (**F**); right seminal vesicle (**G**—not shown); left seminal vesicle (**H**—not shown); excision margin of right ureter (**J**—not shown); excision margin of left ureter (**K**—not shown); lymph nodes in right perivesical fat (**L**); lymph nodes in left perivesical fat (**M** —not shown).

128b

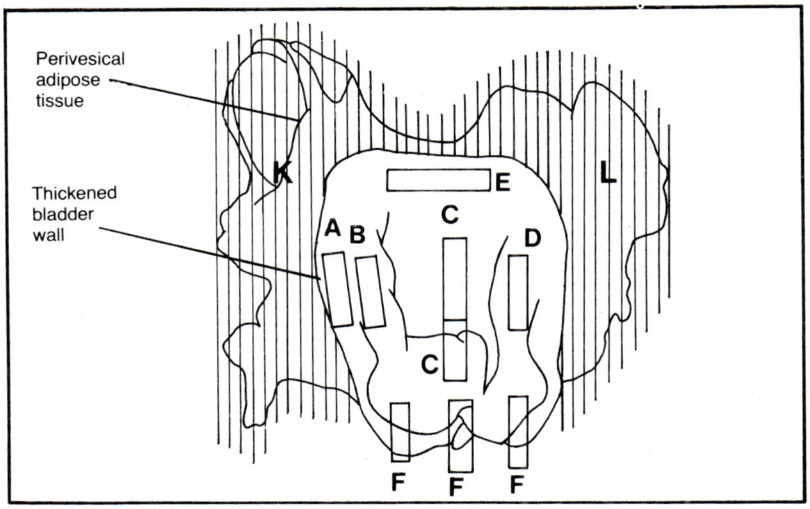

CHAPTER 7
RESPIRATORY SYSTEM

Small specimens

The most frequent biopsy from the lungs and pleura is obtained by biopsy needle or forceps, percutaneously or via a bronchoscope or mediastinoscope. Small biopsies can be taken for the investigation of diffuse lung shadowing, pulmonary and pleural masses and pleural effusions. The specimens are tiny and impossible to orientate; they are embedded whole and serially sectioned. In some departments these biopsies are fixed in Bouin's solution. This results in better preservation of nuclear morphology, and the increase in hardness of the fixed tissue is seldom a problem with these tiny fragments. The description can be short, for example, 'A small pale irregular tissue fragment measuring . . . . All embedded'.

Large specimens

Large specimens comprise open lung biopsies taken for diagnosis as above, and lobulectomies, lobectomies, pneumonectomies and resections of pleura performed for the treatment of tumours and inflammatory conditions such as bronchiectasis and pleurisy.

Dissection of specimen

Lung

In some specialist departments, lobectomy and pneumonectomy specimens are inflated with fixative before dissection, but in most routine laboratories the specimens are fixed simply by immersion in formalin.

Before dissection, the specimen should be measured and weighed, and the external surface examined and described (**129, 130**). Particular attention should be given to the hilum if this is present.

In all cases of neoplasia, the resection lines of the bronchus and pulmonary vessels should be blocked, and the hilar lymph nodes removed before the specimen is dissected further (**130b**). The larger airways are then opened with fine scissors to try to establish the site of origin and extent of involvement of a tumour. If the origin of the tumour from a large bronchus is obvious, blocks can be taken longitudinally along the bronchus into the tumour. In many cases the origin is more difficult to establish, and close parallel cuts are then best made through the tumour at right angles to the main bronchi to the area (**130b, 131a**). Blocks are taken from the centre and periphery of the tumour, from bronchi adjacent to the tumour even if they do not seem macroscopically involved, and from the overlying pleura (**131b**).

In lobulectomy specimens or where there is a small peripheral tumour large bronchi may not be present, and more information can be gained from close cuts through the specimen at right angles to the visceral pleura (**132**).

The condition of the lung distal to the tumour and also well away from the tumour should be noted. Cuts should be made through the specimen either transversely or coronally, and blocks taken to look for tumour spread, bronchiectasis, endogenous lipid pneumonia, bacterial infection, diffuse fibrosing conditions or other pulmonary disease which might be bilateral.

In non-neoplastic specimens (taken, for example, for bronchiectasis (**133, 134, 135**) scarring or hamartoma), it is not necessary to take resection margins, although blocks should be taken from large bronchi. If a focal lesion is present, sampling can be based on principles similar to those for neoplastic specimens. Diffuse pathology can be displayed by coronal or sagittal slicing (**135**). Blocks are taken from focal lesions, and from each lobe in diffuse disease. If bronchiectasis is found, special stains for amyloid (Congo red, thioflavine T) should be requested.

Pleura

Sheets of pleura (**136**) taken for the diagnosis or palliation of mesothelioma or pleurisy are sliced at close intervals at right angles to the pleural surface.

Lung and pleura: Macroscopical report

Type of specimen	Irregular piece of lung, lobulectomy, lobectomy, right or left pneumonectomy, sheet of pleura Other tissues attached to specimen (oesophagus, diaphragm, pericardium)
Measurements	Size and weight of lung specimens Area and thickness of pleural sheets
Description	
Focal lesions	Site, and origin if this can be established (subpleural, hilar, upper pole of lung, from main bronchus, from visceral pleura); size; growth pattern (intraluminal, diffuse and ill-defined, local with 'pushing' edges); colour; consistency (soft, necrotic, firm and fibrous) Relation to other tissues (pleura, oesophagus, pericardium, diaphragm)
Rest of specimen	*Bronchi* Colour; size (normal, dilated); condition of walls (thickened, friable, calcified) *Lung parenchyma* Colour; consistency (oedematous, consolidated, gritty, nodular); presence of bronchopneumonia, lobar pneumonia, secondary bronchiectasis *Pleura* Colour; consistency; contour
Other tissues	Number, size and cut-surface appearances of hilar and other lymph nodes Appearance of oesophagus, etc., to record any abnormality other than the tumour involvement described above

Example 129-131

The specimen is a lobe of lung measuring 17 × 12 x 4.5 cm and weighing 325 g. At the apex the pleural surface is discoloured and distorted. Below this there is a firm white tumour mass approximately 6 cm in diameter, its outline irregular but clearly demarcated from the adjacent lung parenchyma. The tumour extends up to but not through the overlying visceral pleura. The large bronchi in the specimen are not involved by tumour, and the lung parenchyma away from the area shows no significant abnormality. The bronchus and vessels at the excision margin appear macroscopically normal. Three lymph nodes ranging from 0.8 to 1 cm in length are present at the hilum.

Blocks

- **A** bronchial resection line × 1
- **B** vascular resection line × 1
- **C** lymph nodes × 3
- **D** tumour × 2
- **E** tumour and adjacent bronchus × 1
- **F** tumour and overlying pleura × 2
- **G** tumour and adjacent lung × 1
- **H** lung away from tumour × 1

129

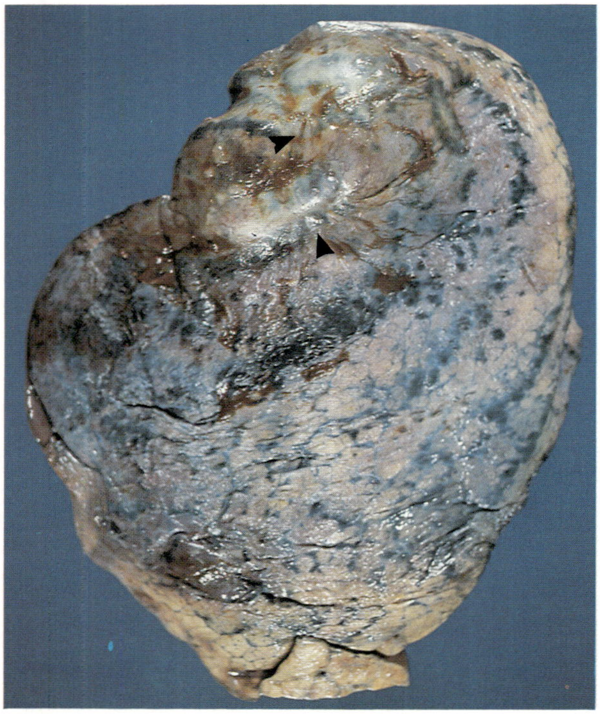

129 The pleural aspect of a lobectomy specimen, removed for carcinoma of the bronchus. Puckering of the visceral pleura (▶) is present over the carcinoma. The firm white tumour tissue can be seen where the carcinoma infiltrates close below the surface.

130a

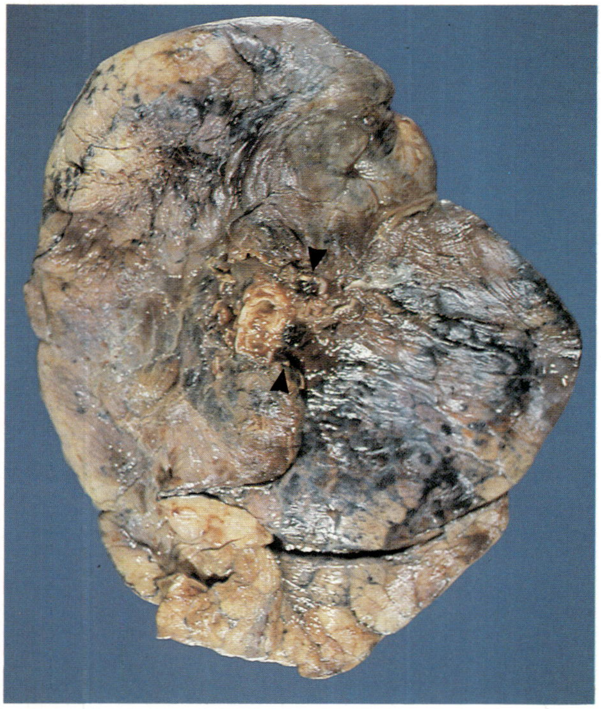

130a The hilar (medial) surface of 129. Small dark lymph nodes are present around the bronchus (▶). There is no macroscopical evidence of the tumour at the bronchial resection margin.

13

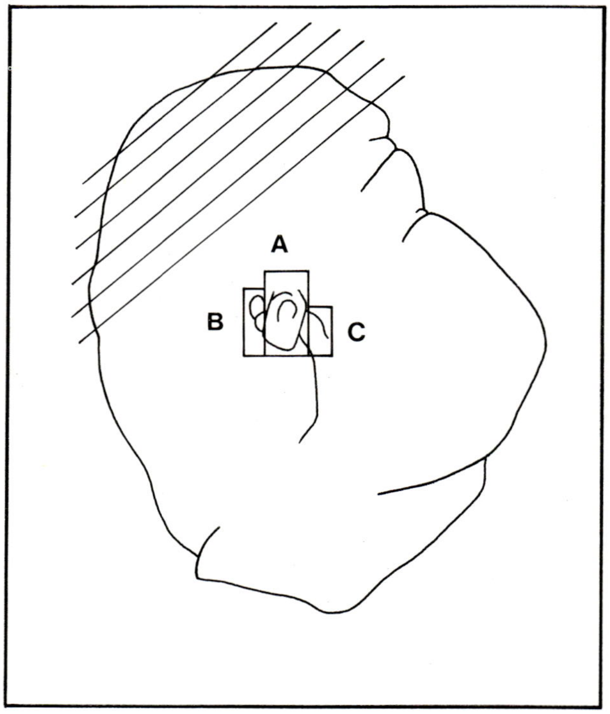

130b Blocks taken from lobectomy or pneumonectomy specimens which contain a tumour, Part 1 (for Part 2, see **131b**): blocks are taken from the bronchial (**A**) and vascular (**B**) excision margins, and from the hilar lymph nodes (**C**). Parallel cuts are then made into the area of the palpable tumour at right angles to the main bronchi to that part of the lung.

131a **A cut slice of the lobectomy specimen 129.** The relations between the tumour, the lung parenchyma and the pleura can be assessed from the slice.

131a

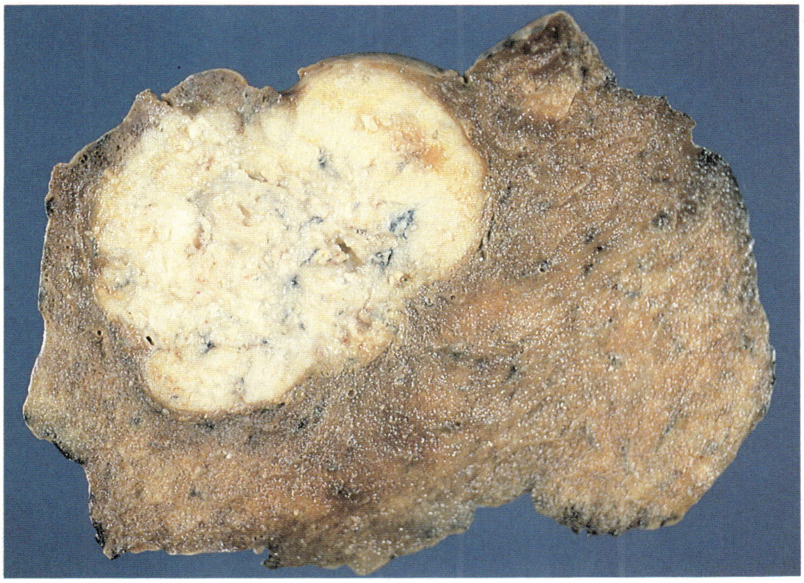

131b **Blocks taken from a lobectomy or pneumonectomy specimen** which contains a tumour, Part 2: centre of tumour (**D**); tumour and adjacent bronchus (**E**); tumour and overlying pleura (**F**); tumour and adjacent lung (**G**); lung away from the tumour (**H**).

131b

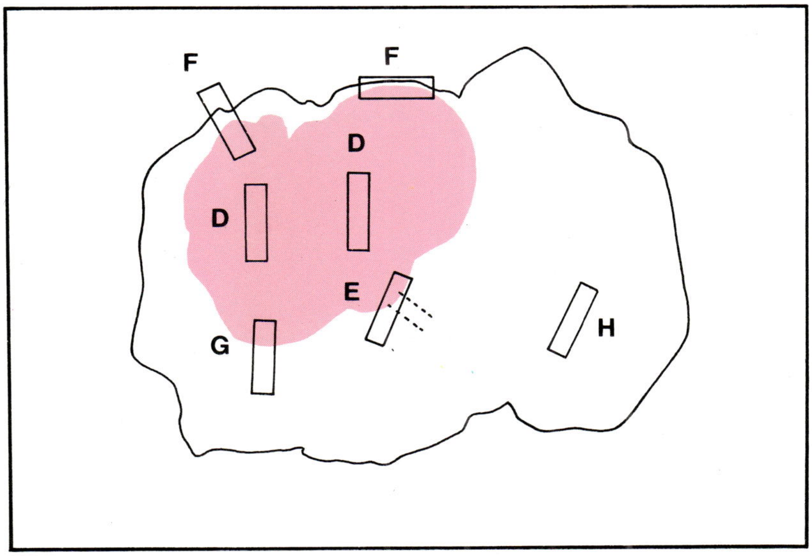

132 **The cut surface of a lobulectomy specimen** containing a well-defined, variegated yellow, pink and red tumour mass. On microscopic examination, this was found to be a metastasis from a renal parenchymal cell carcinoma.

132

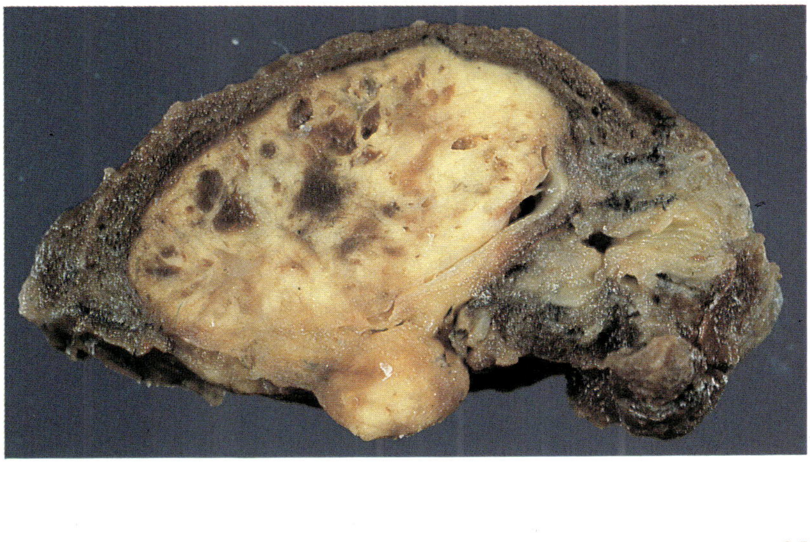

133 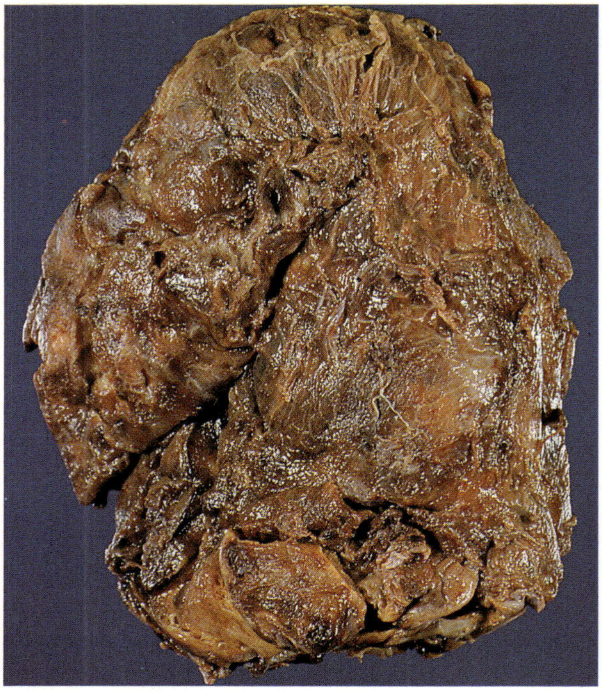

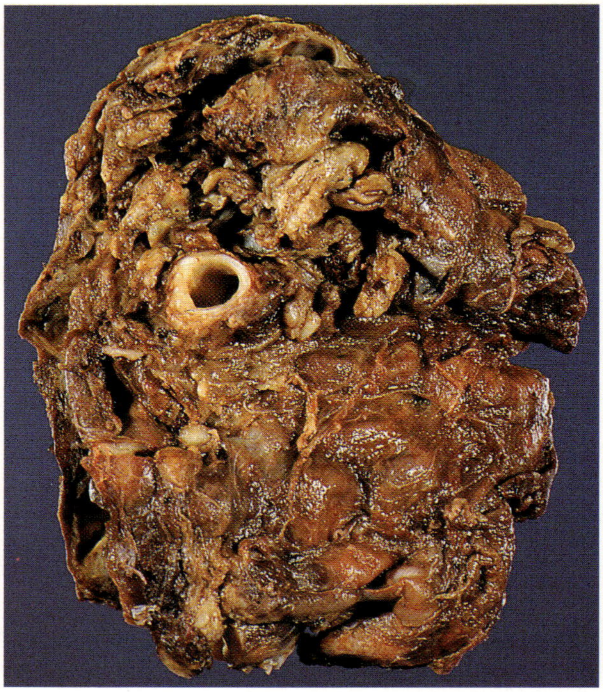 13

135 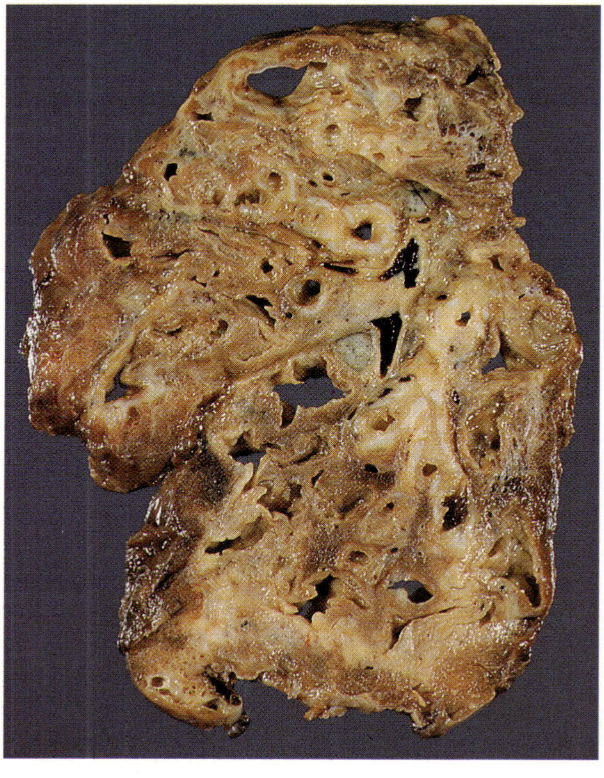

133 and 134 The medial and lateral aspects of a lobectomy specimen removed because of bronchiectasis. The pleural surface is thickened and shows several fine adhesions.

135 The same specimen as 133 and 134 cut coronally. There is dilatation and gross thickening of the bronchi characteristic of bronchiectasis, with loss and distortion of the adjacent parenchyma.

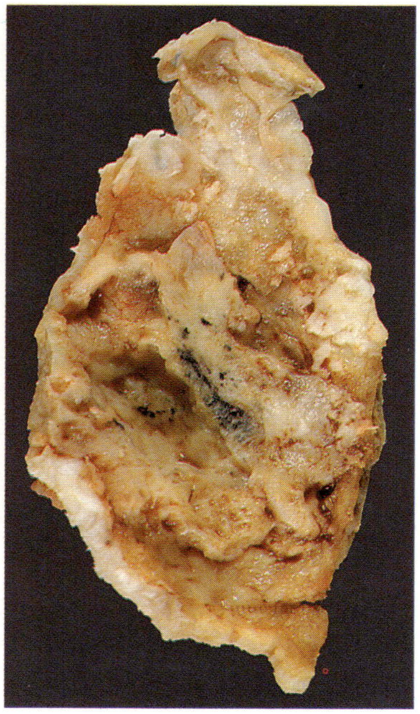 136

136 A sheet of diffusely thickened parietal pleura. This was found on microscopic examination to be caused by chronic pleurisy.

CHAPTER 8
SKIN

Small skin biopsies may be superficial scrapings, shavings of the surface of an exophytic lesion, punch biopsies or small ellipses taken to diagnose inflammatory and degenerative conditions, cysts, hamartomas, dysplasias and neoplasms. Larger ellipses or irregular sheets of skin are excised for the treatment of pilonidal sinus and skin tumours.

Scrapings and other irregular fragments are embedded whole. Punch biopsies are usually bisected through the epidermis and underlying tissues, and both halves are embedded. If a vesicle is present on the biopsy it should be preserved intact if possible and the specimen embedded whole, so that the lesion is cut only after it has the support of the embedding wax (**137**). This is not possible with large bullae, and in these cases sections from the periphery of the lesion should be blocked (**138**). Intradermal cysts should be bisected, and half or both pieces embedded (**139, 140**).

There are several methods for taking blocks from an ellipse of skin bearing a tumour. The main purpose is to diagnose the tumour type and establish how close it is to the lateral and deep excision margins. The standard method for sampling small skin ellipses is to make a cut through the specimen transversely at the point where the tumour appears to be nearest to the lateral excision margin (**141a, 141b**). Either both parts can be embedded, or parallel cuts can be made to produce further blocks.

With larger skin specimens, the deep and lateral excision margins may be painted with India ink so that it is easy to establish whether a sinus or a neoplasm has been completely excised. Transverse, cruciate or radial blocks are taken again through those points where the tumour appears to come closest to the lateral excision margin (**142a, 142b, 143a, 143b**).

An ellipse of skin and subcutis containing a pilonidal sinus should be cut transversely at close intervals at right angles to the skin surface, and blocks taken to demonstrate the sinus and its relation with the skin and subcutis.

Skin: Macroscopical report	
Site	Site of the biopsy or excision should be recorded
Type of specimen	Curettings, irregular fragments, punch biopsy cylinder, ellipse, irregular sheet
Measurements	Maximum dimension of small specimens Aggregate of fragments Size of tissue as area of skin surface and depth of subcutaneous tissue ('An ellipse of skin measuring 3.1 cm × 5.3 cm with underlying tissue to a depth of 0.2 cm')
Description	
Focal lesion	Size (area or diameter); height above the skin surface and extension into the dermis Colour; contour (rounded, bossed, vesicular, bullous, irregular); consistency (firm, rubbery, hard, friable); texture (granular, glossy, ulcerated, papillary) Distance from nearest excision margins
Rest of skin	Colour; texture

Example 142a-143a
An irregular piece of skin measuring 7 × 6.1 cm, with underlying tissue to a depth of 2.7 cm. It contains a firm, nodular tumour 3 cm in diameter, with a crusted, ulcerated surface which is raised above the level of the surrounding epidermis to a height of 0.6 cm. The cut surface of the tumour shows ill-defined areas of red and white tissue infiltrating through the dermis and subcutis as far as the deep excision line.

Blocks
A tumour with deep resection margin × 2
B tumour with lateral resection margin × 1
C tumour and adjacent skin × 2

137
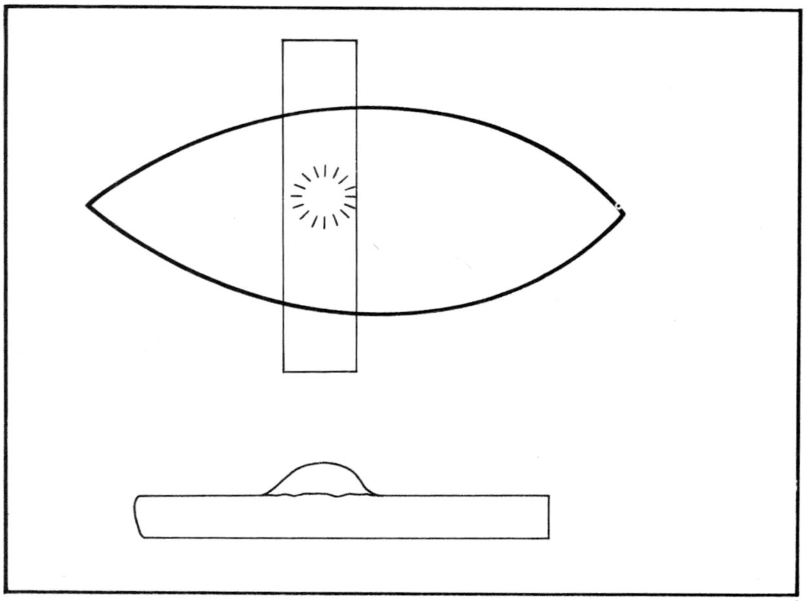

137 Block taken from a small vesicle or bulla of the skin.

138
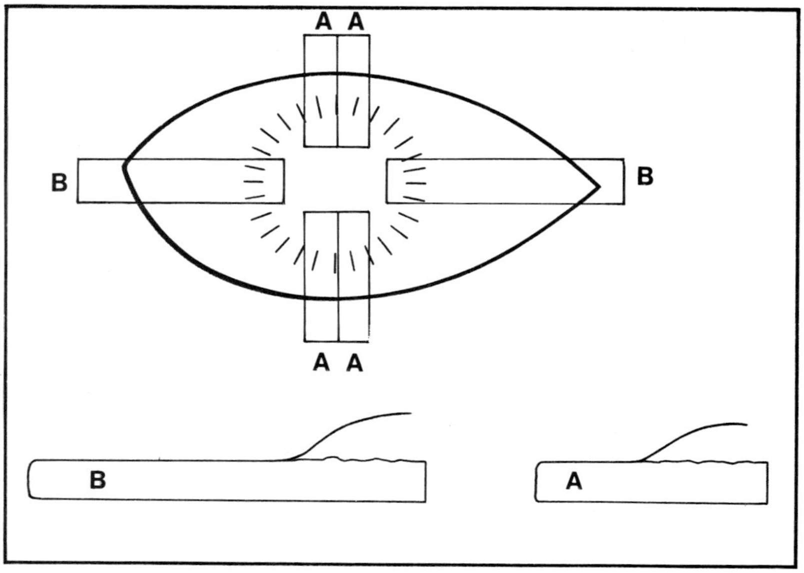

138 Blocks taken from a large vesicle or bulla of the skin: bulla and closest excision margin (**A**); bulla and furthest excision margin (**B**).

139 An ellipse of pale hair-bearing skin with a smooth-surfaced, ovoid intradermal nodule.

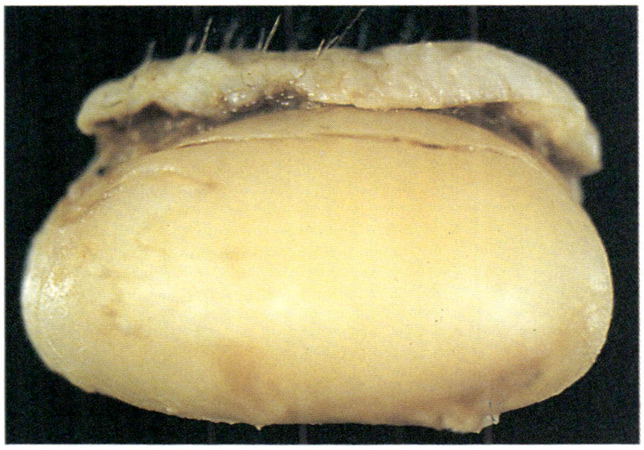

139

140 The nodule in 139 shown on section to be cystic. The lumen contains yellow putty-like material (in which, in this case, there is focal calcification). This is the typical appearance of a pilar cyst.

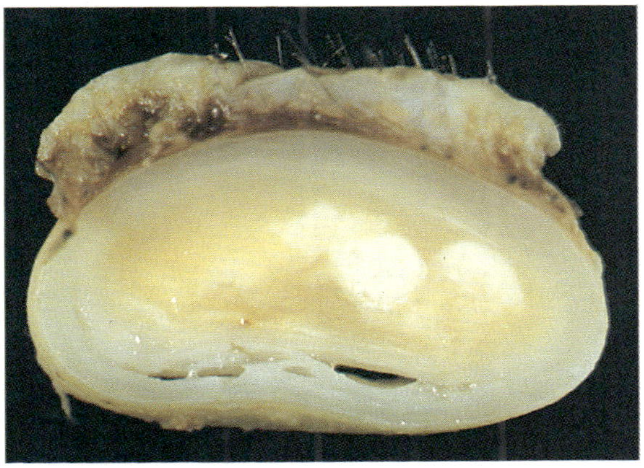

140

141a A small ellipse of pale skin containing a slightly raised, irregular pigmented lesion which is just clear of one lateral excision margin.

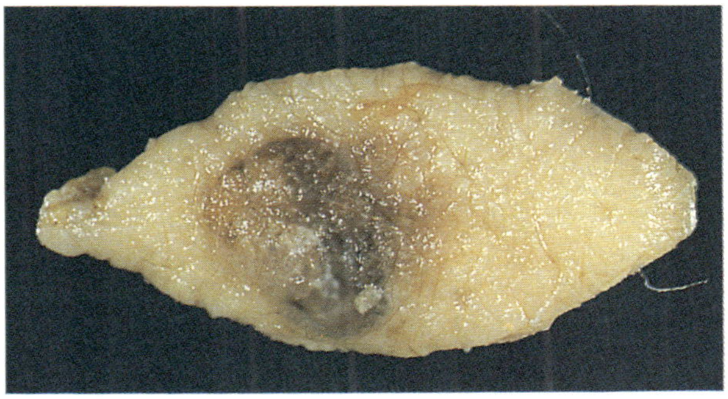

141a

141b Blocks taken from a small ellipse of skin containing a tumour. The first cut made through the lesion comes as close as possible to the nearest excision margin (▶). Further cuts are made parallel to this and the slices containing tumour are embedded. The face revealed by the first cut is embedded so that it is sectioned first when histological slides are being prepared.

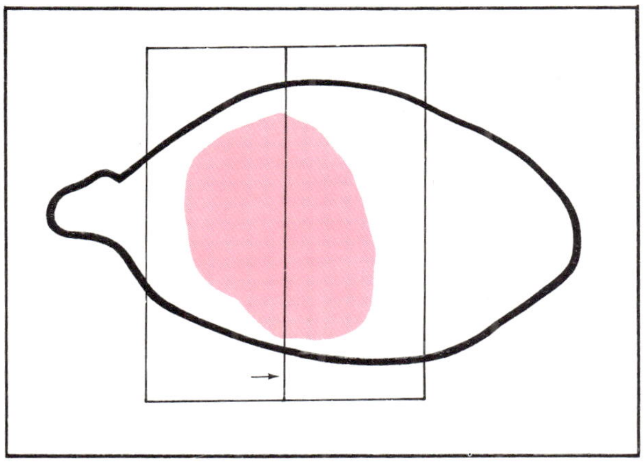

141b

142a

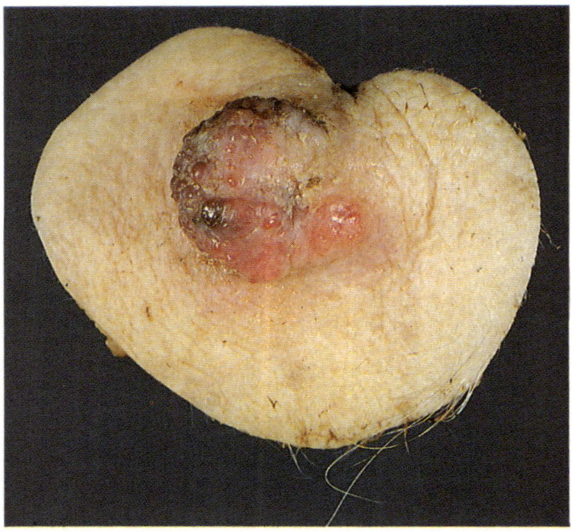

142a A raised nodular pink tumour mass on an irregular sheet of skin.

142b

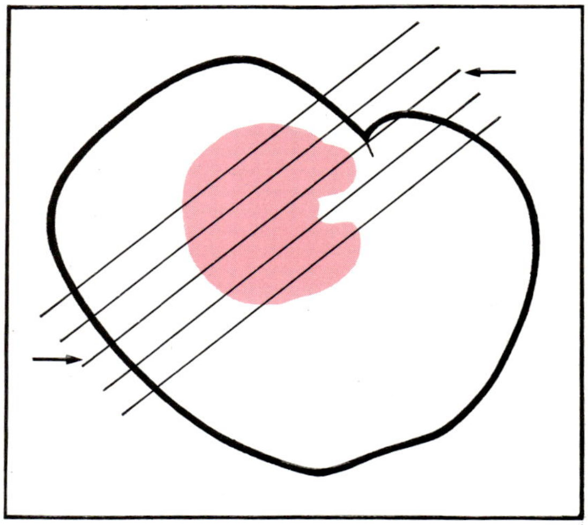

142b Transverse incisions through 142a. The first cut should pass through the lateral excision nearest to the tumour (▶).

143a

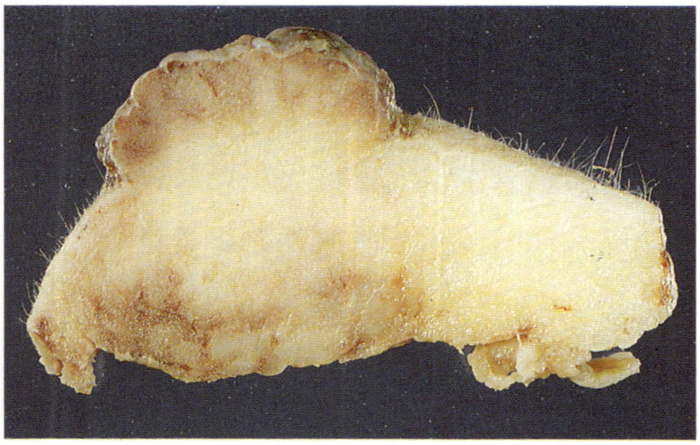

143a A section of 142a showing that the tumour infiltrates deeply into the dermis and subcutis. Histologically this was found to be a Merkel cell tumour (neuroendocrine tumour of skin).

14

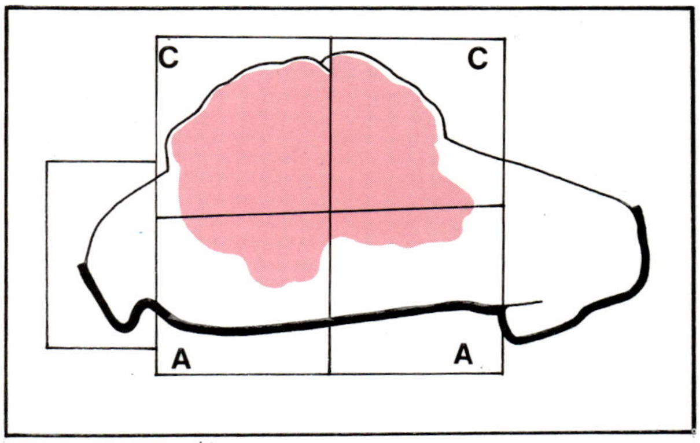

143b Blocks taken from a large skin specimen containing a tumour. These are taken from the slices which shows the lateral excision margin nearest to the tumour. Tumour and deep excision margin (**A**); lateral excision margin nearest tumour (**B**); tumour and adjacent skin (**C**); skin away from tumour (**D**—not shown).

CHAPTER 9
LYMPHORETICULAR SYSTEM

Lymph nodes

Lymph nodes are excised specifically, rather than as part of a resection specimen, for a variety of conditions. Probably the commonest is cryptogenic lymph node enlargement, which may be due to reactive hyperplasia, specific infections, lymphoma or metastatic carcinoma. Where possible the tissue should be sent unfixed to the laboratory.

Needle biopsies are sometimes performed on nodes that are thought to contain metastatic carcinoma, especially when the patient is too ill to withstand lymphadenectomy. Diagnosis and typing of lymphoma is based on a combination of cellular and architectural features. These can be very difficult to diagnose on a needle core, and removal of an entire node should be recommended.

Dissection of specimen

Specimens thought to be infective should have one half of the fresh, unfixed biopsy sent in a dry, sterile container for microbiological examination.

In cases of suspected lymphoma, as soon as possible after excision the node should be bisected through the hilum (**144, 145**) and small pieces of tissue taken for preservation in liquid nitrogen for immunocytochemical staining. In addition, in some departments imprints are made on clean dry microscope slides before the node is immersed in formalin. These imprints allow better assessment of the cytology of the constituent cells and enable special stains such as Giemsa to be used more easily. The remaining node is then fixed in formalin. If the node is large, further cuts parallel to the initial incision are made, so that diffusion of the fixative is not delayed by the fibrous capsule of the node.

If the node is received in formalin, it should be bisected or sliced if necessary to ensure good fixation. After fixation, if the cut surface of the node is homogeneous, a block from the centre is taken. With larger specimens and those where focal lesions are present, several blocks may be necessary. Where processing into resin is intended, pieces of tissue no more than 3 mm thick should be submitted.

The dissection of lymph nodes from specimens resected for carcinoma of the breast, gastrointestinal tract, etc. is described on p15.

Lymph nodes: Macroscopical report

Site	Site of origin of the lymph node or nodes (cervical, paraaortic, etc)
Type of specimen	Needle biopsy, lymph node, mass of adipose tissue containing nodes
Measurements	Size of adipose or other tissue mass in which nodes are included, if present Number of nodes (under measurement) and greatest diameter of node or nodes
Description	If multiple, whether the nodes are discrete or matted together Appearance of cut surface (uniformity, colour, nodularity)

144

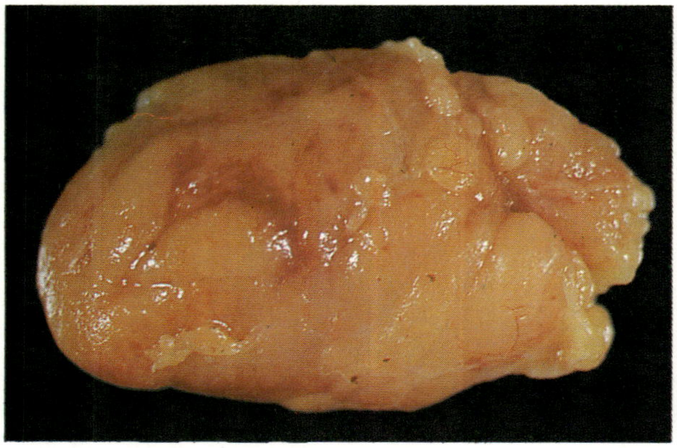

144 **The external aspect of a lymph node** showing a smooth, lobulated capsular surface.

145

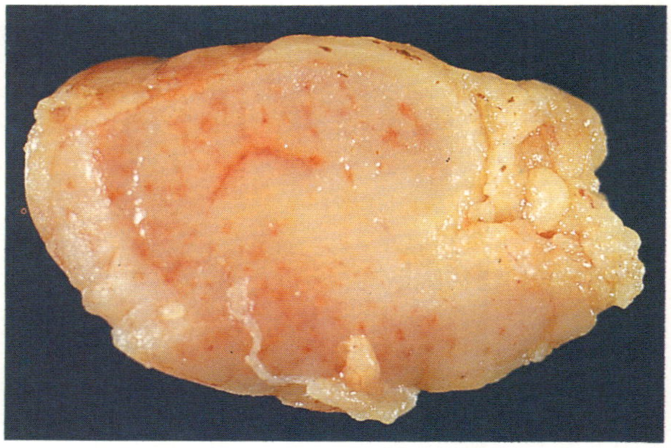

145 **The cut surface of 144** showing pale pink tissue with a prominent vascular pattern. On microscopic examination the node was found to be replaced by lymphoplasmacytoid lymphoma.

Spleen

Splenectomy may be performed because of traumatic rupture, lymphoproliferative and myeloproliferative diseases, hypersplenism from other causes and as part of a gastrectomy procedure.

Dissection of specimen

Even after several hours of immersion in formalin, intact spleens are often unfixed in the centre of the specimen. On receipt, they should be weighed and measured, and sliced at about 1 cm intervals from the hilar surface towards the capsule. Either the capsule can be left intact so that the slices are kept in sequence (**146, 147**) (and absorbent paper inserted between the slices to aid further fixation), or it is cut through and the slices laid out in order (**148, 149, 150**).

If the specimen has been received fresh, after slicing as above, tissue for freezing or imprints can be taken if necessary.

After fixation, the cut surface of the specimen should be examined. Malphigian bodies can normally be seen scattered uniformly through the parenchyma, and may be prominent in lymphoproliferative disorders. Where there is diffuse disease (**150**), at least four random blocks should be taken. Where focal lesions are present (**148**), blocks are taken from then and from the junction with the surrounding parenchyma. The splenic hilum should be examined for nodules which might be lymph nodes (**147**), splenunculi or pancreatic tissue, and these should also be blocked.

Splenectomy: Macroscopical report

Type of specimen	Spleen, splenunculus; other tissues attached
Measurements	Weight, size Size of focal lesion
Description	
Outer surface	Colour; contour (bosselated, ruptured, elongated, nodular); consistency (soft and diffluent, firm, friable, hard); texture (capsular thickening, covering of fibrin or blood clot)
Cut surface	Colour; uniformity (mottled with tiny white areas, focal pale pink patches, prominent vascular pattern)
Other lesions	Presence of splenunculi, nodes; invasion by tumour from pancreas, large bowel

Example 146-148

The specimen consists of a spleen weighing 245 g and measuring 14 × 8 × 5 cm. The capsule is smooth and shiny. The cut surface shows numerous yellow lobulated nodules, ranging from 0.2-2.3 cm in diameter. Elsewhere the splenic parenchyma appears unremarkable.

Blocks

- **A** focal nodules × 3
- **B** blocks from hilar surface × 1
- **C** blocks from lateral capsular surface × 1

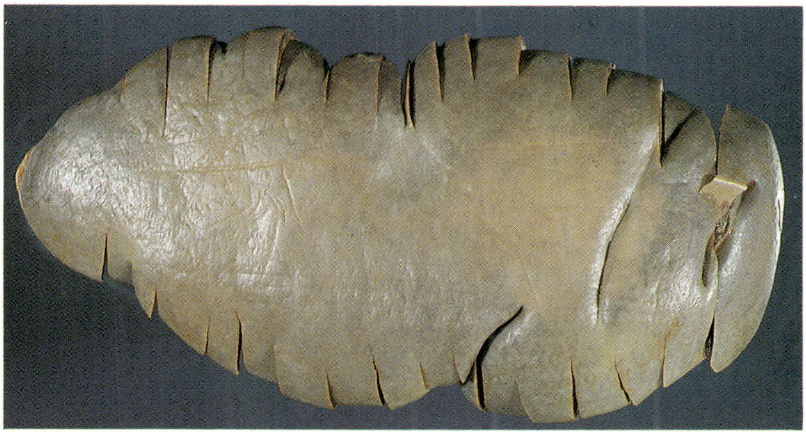

146 **An enlarged spleen** from a patient with non-Hodgkins' lymphoma. The capsular surface is smooth and shiny.

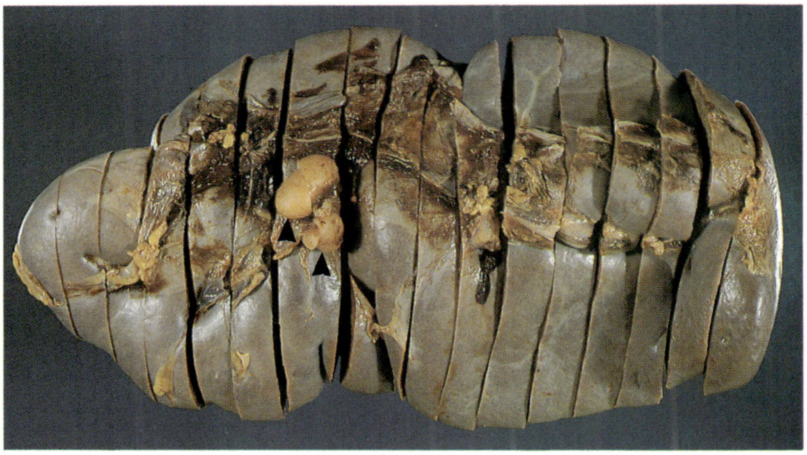

147 **The medial aspect of 146** showing two yellowish ovoid lymph nodes at the splenic hilum (▶). The spleen has been sliced from the hilar surface almost through to the capsular surface, leaving the latter intact to keep the slices in sequence. Absorbent paper can be inserted between the leaves and the specimen left to fix further.

148

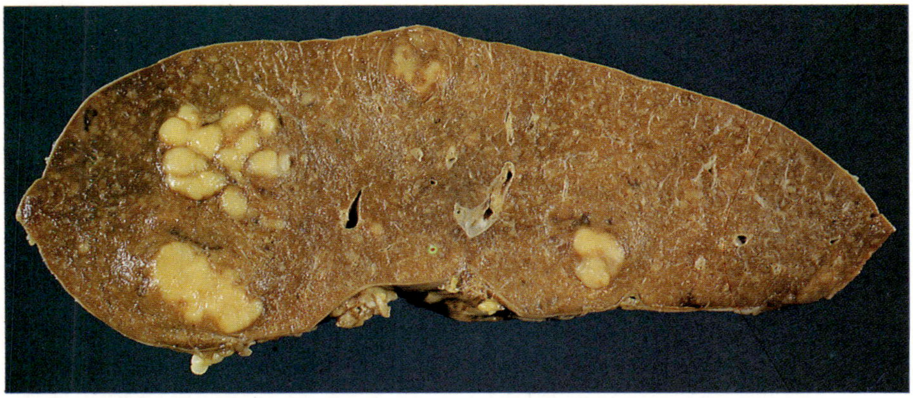

148 A separated slice from 147. The cut surface shows several well-defined areas of lobulated yellow lymphoma tissue.

149

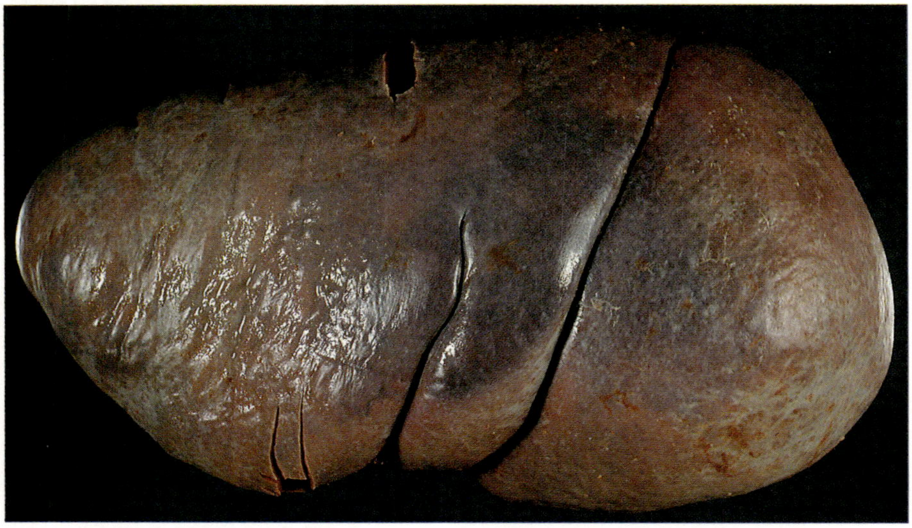

149 The spleen from a patient with hairy cell leukaemia. The specimen was received unfixed and tissue was taken for freezing and imprints.

150

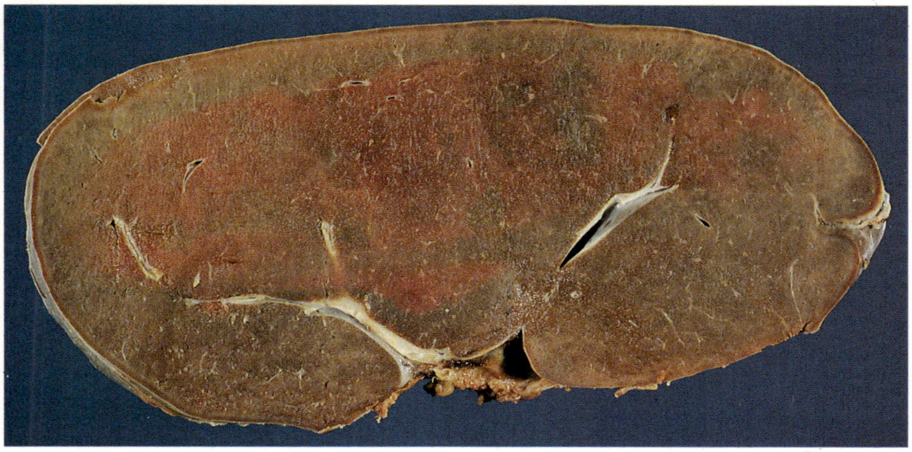

150 Specimen 149 sliced through and laid out in a shallow tray to fix. The cut surface has a homogeneous red-brown appearance; no malphigian bodies or focal lesions are apparent.

Bone marrow

Trephine biopsies of bone marrow from the iliac crest are taken to investigate haematological disorders and metastatic carcinoma. They usually consist of small cores of hard brown tissue, and are submitted intact for decalcification and processing. The length, diameter and colour of the tissue should be recorded on the macroscopical report.

If the tissue is to be stained with methyl green pyronin stain, decalcification should be in EDTA rather than formic acid, and the length of time in the decalcification fluid should be as short as possible.

Thymus

Thymectomy may be performed in the treatment of myasthenia gravis, for cysts and for neoplasms such as thymoma, teratoma and lymphoma. The tissue received varies in size from a few irregular fragments to a large nodular mass (**151, 152**). The specimen should be measured and, if intact rather than fragmented, the excision margins should be identified and can be marked with India ink. Large specimens are sliced with close parallel cuts through the tissue and the cut surface is examined.

Blocks are taken from any focal lesion or variegated areas, if present, and from the excision margins. Numerous blocks are taken from the walls of cysts to try to establish their histogenesis. If the tissue is homogeneous, several pieces from the periphery and centre should be submitted. Fragments are embedded in their entirety.

Example 151-152

The specimen is a partial thymectomy consisting of an ovoid mass of rubbery grey and purple tissue 5.5 cm in diameter and 8.7 cm long, to which is attached an irregular extension measuring 1.2 × 1.5 × 1.6 cm. The cut surface shows that the mass is cystic. The wall is uniform, measures 0.4 cm thick, and the lumen contains soft friable brown material. The other tissue present, in the extension of the specimen, is soft and white and appears encapsulated.

Blocks

A	cyst wall × 5
B	other tissue × 2

Thymus: Macroscopical report

Type of specimen	Irregular fragments, tissue mass, partial or total thymectomy specimen
Measurements	Dimensions in three planes, or aggregate volume of fragments Size of focal lesions
Description	
Fragments	'Several irregular brown fragments . . .'
Large specimens	*External surface* Colour; contour (nodular, irregular, adherent to surrounding tissues) *Cut surface* Focal lesions (appearance, size and relation to excision margins); rest of gland (uniform, cystic, nodular, gritty)

151

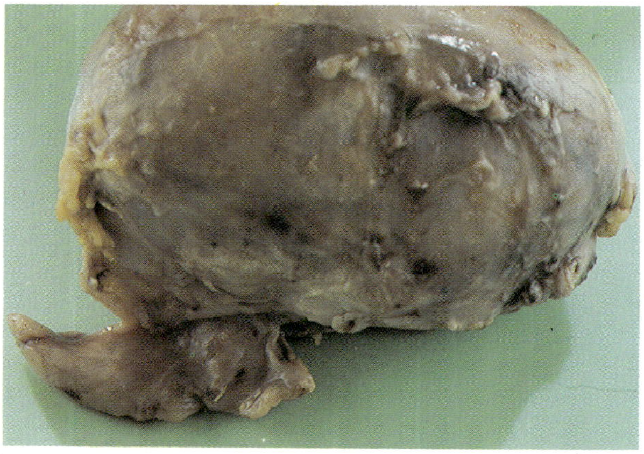

151 Part of an enlarged thymus containing a smooth-surfaced mass.

152

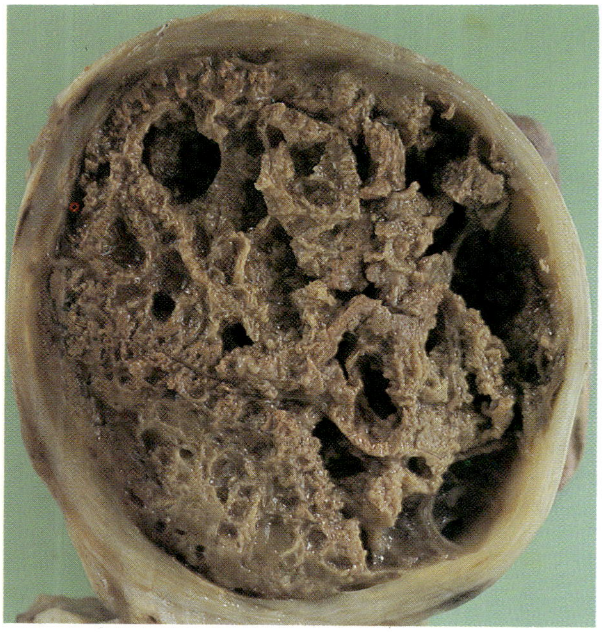

152 A section of 151 showing that the mass is cystic. It has a thick wall of firm white tissue and contains soft friable brown material. (Numerous sections from the cyst wall were examined under the microscope, but the histogenesis of the cyst was not evident.)

CHAPTER 10
ENDOCRINE SYSTEM

Pituitary gland

Pituitary tumours may be removed trans-sphenoidally by curettage and/or aspiration, or transfrontally by dissection or curettage. All curettage fragments should be blocked, including blood clots, and the contents of the aspirator (to which formalin has been added in theatre or in the laboratory) should be carefully sieved to retrieve small fragments of tissue.

The macroscopical report is usually limited to a short description and aggregate measurement, for example 'Several irregular red and brown fragments together measuring . . .'.

Adrenal gland

Small specimens

Small biopsies of the adrenal glands are very rarely taken. Ectopic adrenal cortical tissue is sometimes encountered, and the commonest surgical specimen of adrenal tissue in many hospitals is probably a nodule of ectopic adrenal cortex discovered incidentally at herniorrhaphy or laparotomy. These are small, rounded yellow nodules which can be measured and described, and then bisected or embedded whole.

Large specimens

Adrenal cortical tumours are rare. Adenomas represent the most frequent specimens from the adrenal gland. In these cases, and for the rarer adrenal carcinomas and medullary tumours, the whole adrenal gland is excised. The size and weight of the specimen should be recorded, as these measurements have a direct bearing on the diagnosis and prognosis. Adenomas rarely exceed 50 g or a diameter of 5 cm, and it is unwise to regard large adrenal neoplasms over 100 g as definitely benign, even in the absence of histological features of malignancy. Adrenal cortical carcinomas present late and can weigh 500 g or more.

Adrenal medullary tumours are also rare. Neuroblastoma and ganglioneuroblastoma arise in children and form large, soft grey masses with areas of haemorrhage and necrosis. Ganglioneuroma, the counterpart in young adults, is smaller, pale, homogeneous and firm because of the fibrous stroma which develops in and around these tumours. Phaeochromocytomas are found principally in adults, and also grow to large masses. On the cut surface they are soft, haemorrhagic and yellow, grey or red-brown (**153, 154, 155**).

Bilateral adrenalectomy is performed occasionally for the palliation of the effects of ectopic ACTH-secreting tumours when the primary tumour cannot be found. The operation was once commonly performed for the palliation of breast carcinoma.

Dissection of specimen

If the specimen is received fresh and a diagnosis of phaeochromocytoma is suspected or established, a block-sized piece should be taken for dichromate fixation. The process requires fresh tissue, which is placed directly into dichromate fixative (formalin fixation allows diffusion of catecholamines into the fixative and subsequent treatment with dichromate can result in a negative reaction). The chromaffin reaction depends on the ability of catecholamines to reduce dichromate solution to insoluble coloured adenochrome pigments (noradrenalin gives a weaker reaction than adrenaline). The tissue can then be processed and sectioned, when the catecholamines appear as brown granules within the tumour cells. The reaction is not of practical use nowadays (except for the histological demonstration of these granules) since hormone estimation on serum or fresh tissue extracts provides more reliable data on the types of catecholamines produced by the tumour.

Attached to the adrenal there may be tissues such as kidney, liver, and posterior abdominal wall muscle. These should be described and their relation to the tumour noted. If the completeness of excision is in doubt and the tumour extends close to an excision margin, the outside of the specimen should be marked with India ink. The specimen is measured and the adrenal gland is separated from the surrounding tissues and weighed. Parallel cuts are then made through the gland and tumour at close intervals. Tissue from focal lesions, the adrenal capsule, the normal gland and the vascular pedicle (if present) should be blocked (**154b**). Invasion of large veins may be evident macroscopically.

Nowadays histopathologists are seldom called upon to determine whether an adrenal neoplasm is functioning – surgery is rarely performed in advance of serum hormone estimations. Nevertheless, a block of non-neoplastic adrenal tissue away from the tumour should be taken to look for atrophy. If atrophy is present, the adenoma is almost certainly secreting glucocorticosteroids (aldosterone and sex hormones do not inhibit pituitary ACTH secretion and have no suppressant effect on the adrenal).

Example 153-155
The specimen consists of a grossly enlarged adrenal gland measuring 9 × 8 × 8.5 cm and weighing 42 g. The normal outline of the adrenal is distorted by a well-circumscribed, lobulated mass measuring approximately 8 cm in diameter. The outer surface is smooth and the capsule appears intact. On examination of the cut surface, the tumour is shown to be composed of soft yellow and white tissue with large areas of recent and old haemorrhage. A small fragment of uninvolved adrenal gland is present at one side of the mass; this has the normal yellow colour and shows no evidence of atrophy.

Blocks

A	central part of tumour × 2
B	tumour and capsule × 5
C	uninvolved adrenal gland × 1

Adrenal gland: Macroscopical report

Type of specimen	Partial adrenalectomy, unilateral adrenalectomy, extended adrenalectomy with nephrectomy and excision of adjacent soft tissues
Measurements	Size and weight Size of focal lesions
Description	
Outer surface	Colour; contour (normal outline of the adrenal still recognizable, distortion by rounded nodules, irregular with extension of tumour through capsule)
Cut surface	*Tumour* Colour (yellow, white, brown, red, variegated with yellow areas, grey areas, etc.); consistency (soft, necrotic, firm, fibrous); contour (circumscribed, irregular) *Rest of gland* Atrophic, pale, nodularity, enlargement
Other tissues	Other tissues present and whether involved by adrenal lesion

153

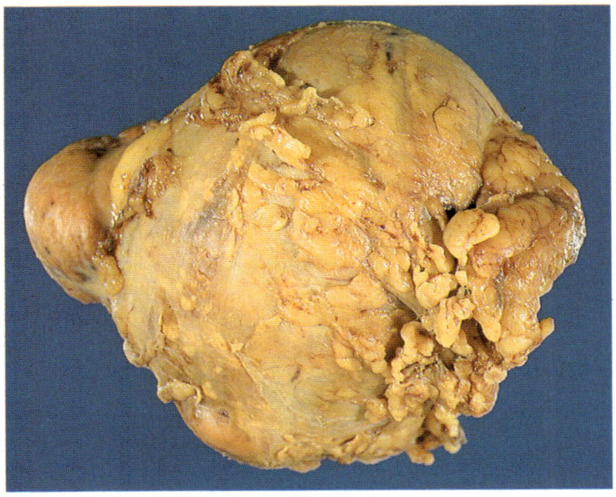

154a

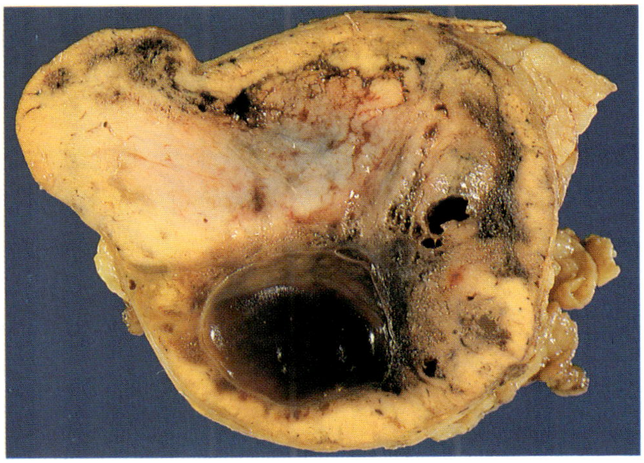

153 A multinodular adrenal tumour. The external surface of the main body of the tumour appears smooth but bears several smaller bosselated tumour masses.

154a The cut surface of the adrenal tumour in 153 which was found on microscopic examination to be a phaeochromocytoma. At least one block should be taken from each macroscopically distinct area of the tumour.

154b

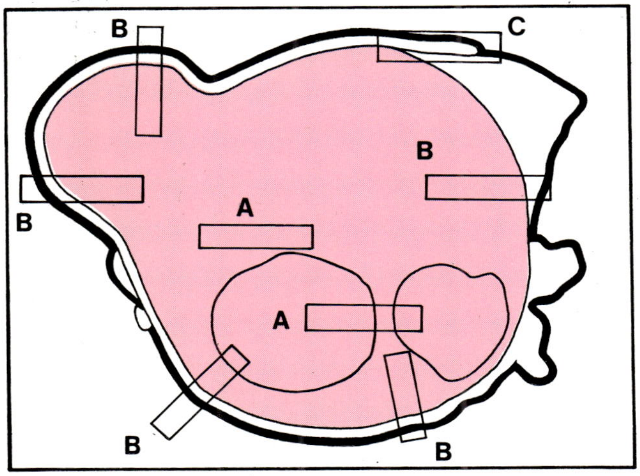

154b Blocks taken from an adrenal tumour: central part of tumour (**A**); tumour and capsule and excision margin (**B**); uninvolved adrenal (**C**).

155 A detail of 154. The non-neoplastic adrenal gland can be seen adjacent to the tumour (▶).

155

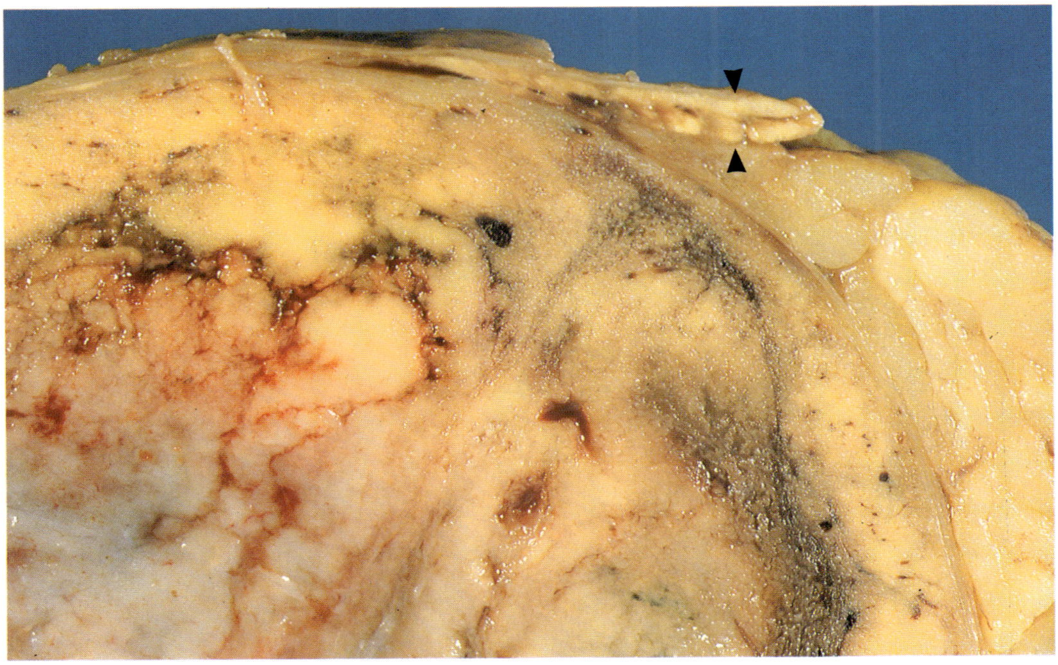

Thyroid gland

Small specimens

The practice of needle aspiration cytology of thyroid nodules is increasing, and is replacing needle biopsy and other small biopsies in the diagnosis of thyroid disease.

Large specimens

Generally speaking, the smallest biopsy specimen received is a thyroid nodule removed with or without the adjacent gland (**156, 157, 158**). A thyroid nodule may be an adenoma, a carcinoma, or a nodule from a multinodular goitre. Rarely, Hashimoto's disease may present as a cold nodule, even though the disease affects the entire gland.

Subtotal thyroidectomy is the commonest large thyroid specimen, and is performed most often for Graves' disease (**159, 160, 161**) and multinodular goitre (**162, 163, 164**). Total thyroidectomy is performed for carcinoma (**165, 166, 167**).

Goitre is a clinical term meaning enlargement of the thyroid, and is seldom used in histopathology reports. Similarly, thyrotoxicosis is a functional term and can be caused by several pathological conditions such as Graves' disease, toxic nodule in a multinodular gland, and adenoma.

Dissection of specimen

The specimen should be weighed, and the dimensions of both lobes and isthmus recorded. The external surface of the gland is described, and the posterior aspect carefully examined for attached parathyroid glands before dissection, as they may otherwise be missed. These brown or yellow-brown ovoid bodies are about 2-3 mm in length. They are usually distinguishable from lymph nodes, which are purple or dark grey from accumulation of carbon particles from the lungs. In practice this distinction is academic, as any small nodule on the surface of a thyroidectomy specimen should be examined histologically. If carcinoma is suspected or proven, the whole surface of the specimen may be marked with India ink before dissection to make it easier to see the relation between the tumour and the excision lines.

The usual method of dissection of a thyroidectomy specimen is to make parallel cuts through the gland. These can be made in the transverse or sagittal plane sequentially through the gland (**160**), and the slices laid out in sequence for further fixation. This method displays the entire gland and its relations with anterior, lateral and posterior structures, but leaves the specimen fragmented. Alternatively, the cuts can be made almost through to the posterior surface; the incisions can then be opened like the pages of a book to demonstrate the pathology present. Cuts should be made as close together as possible to expose small lesions in the gland. This also facilitates the process of taking blocks, as it is possible simply to select sites of interest and trim the cross section to a suitable size.

If the specimen is needed for demonstration or museum purposes, a single coronal section can be made through the entire gland. Blocks can be taken from one half leaving the other intact. The relations of a tumour to the rest of the tissue can usually be adequately assessed, but in cases where there is doubt about the completeness of excision, tumour type or other features of clinical importance, it may be necessary to return to the remaining tissue.

Blocks from all thyroid specimens should include the capsule and excision edges, areas of necrosis or fibrous tissue, and any papillary structures present (**158b**). When numerous blocks are taken it is useful to note their sites on a sketch of the gland, but this is less important if there is obvious diffuse disease.

Solitary nodules should be sampled extensively, especially from the junction of the nodule with the adjacent parenchyma, to assess encapsulation and possible vascular invasion. In multinodular goitre, blocks should be taken from solid white or grey areas to look for malignancy (though in practice this is rare in multinodular thyroids). If calcification or crystallization of colloid is found, the staff responsible for the embedding and section cutting should be warned.

Thyroid: Macroscopical report

Type of specimen	Needle core of thyroid, solitary thyroid nodule, lobe of thyroid, partial, subtotal or total thyroidectomy, extended thyroidectomy with excision of trachea and block dissection of neck
Measurements	Length and diameter of needle core biopsy Size and weight of solitary nodule (diameter if spherical) Size and weight of thyroidectomy specimen (maximum dimensions of the lobes and isthmus)
Description Outer aspect	Colour (purple, red, pink, white, variegated); consistency (rubbery, gelatinous, firm, hard, friable); contour (smooth, nodular, irregular with attached strap muscles); presence of parathyroid glands
Cut surface	*Focal lesion* Diameter of lesion; circumscription and relation to surrounding tissues; cut surface (colour; consistency); presence of papillary structures *Rest of gland* Colour; consistency (dense, beefy, soft, mucoid, hard, friable); contour (lobulated, multinodular, uniform, scarred)
Other tissues	Parathyroid glands, anterior strap muscles of neck

Example 159-161

The specimen consists of a subtotal thyroidectomy weighing 83 g. The right lobe measures 6.3 × 3.5 × 2.9 cm, the left lobe measures 5.9 × 2.9 × 2.5 cm, and the isthmus which is encroached upon by the enlarged lobes measures approximately 1.5 × 0.5 × 0.5 cm. The outer aspect is dark red in colour, and dilated veins run across the capsular surface. The normal lobularity of the gland is accentuated, but there are no distinct nodules. No parathyroid tissue is identified. On sectioning the gland, the cut surface has a mottled brown appearance. No focal lesions are seen.

Blocks

A right lobe × 2
B left lobe × 2
C isthmus × 1

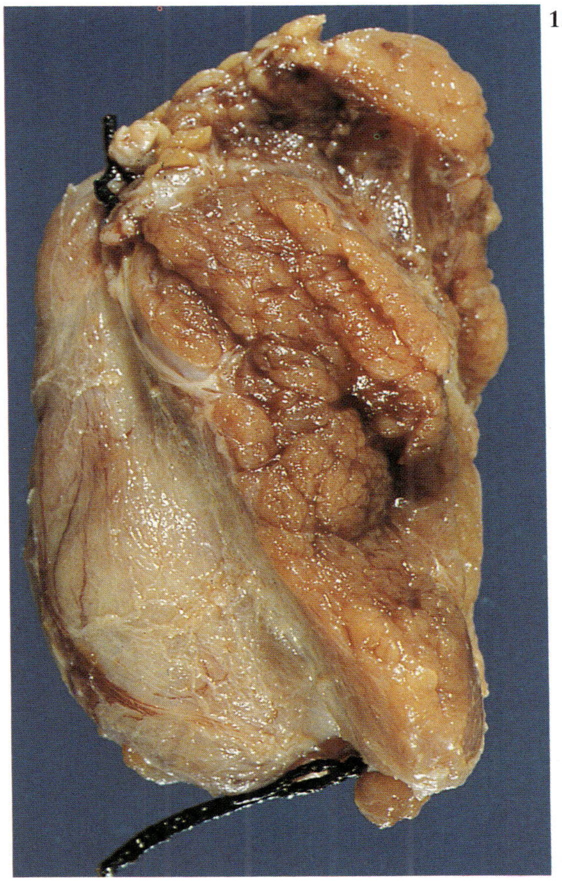

156

156 An excised lobe of thyroid showing the medial resection margin. The surface of the gland has the normal purple-brown colour.

157

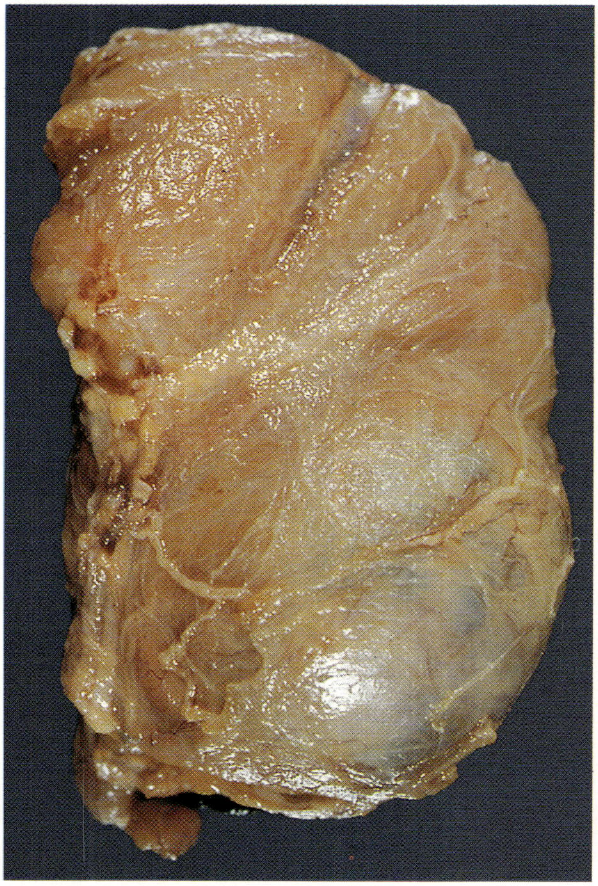

158a

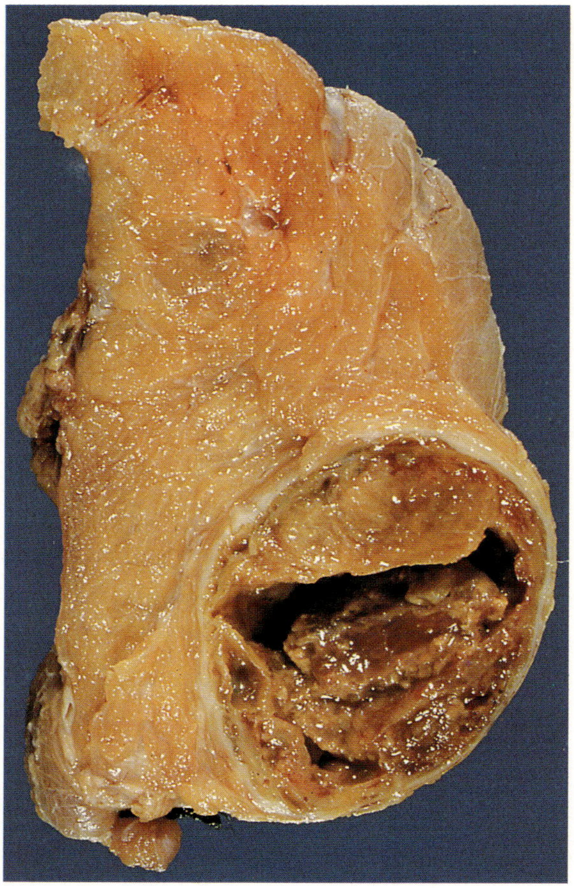

158b

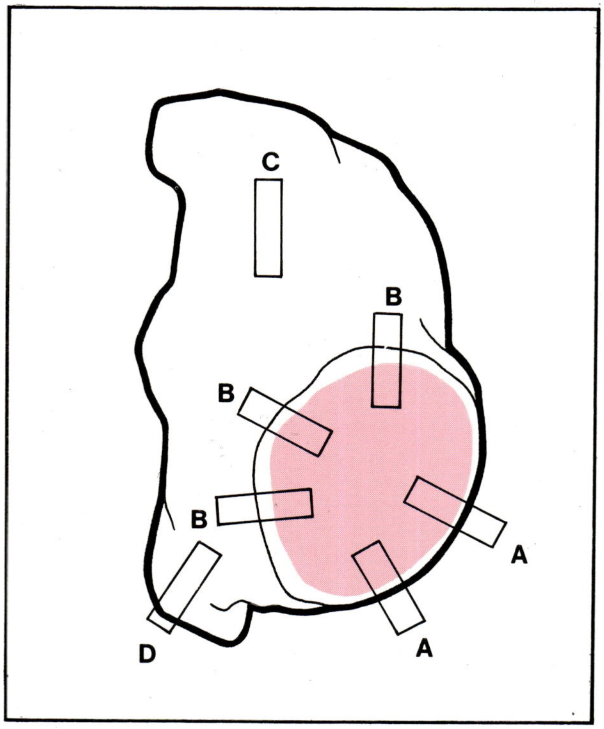

157 The same tissue as 156 from the lateral aspect. At one end of the specimen the thyroid capsule is stretched over a parenchymal nodule which appears slightly darker than the uninvolved gland.

158a The lobe 156 and 157 is shown on section to contain a solitary nodule composed of soft dark-brown tissue with areas of recent haemorrhage. The nodule is well demarcated from the adjacent parenchyma by a distinct white fibrous capsule. The rest of the gland appears normal.

158b Blocks taken from a thyroidectomy specimen containing a focal lesion: lesion and closest excision margin (**A**); lesion and adjacent parenchyma (**B**); unaffected thyroid away from lesion (**C**); isthmus (**D**); and if present, other lobe, lymph nodes and parathyroid glands (not shown).

59

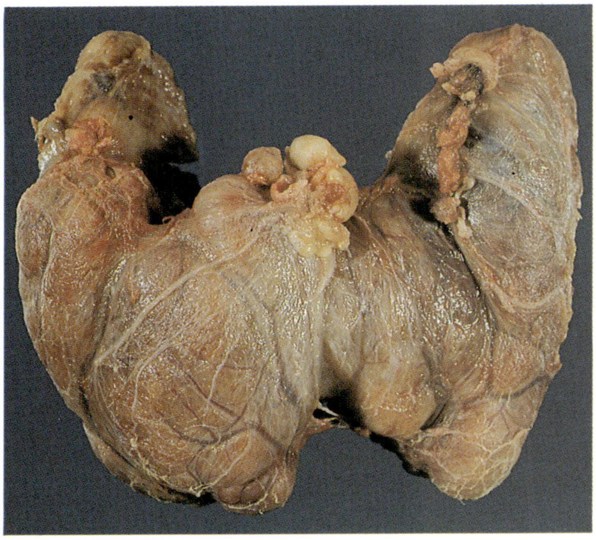

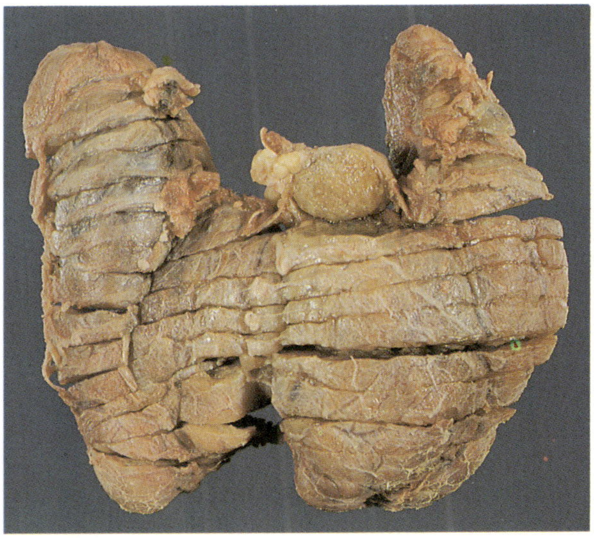

160

159 The external surface of a thyroid from a patient with Graves' disease. The gland is enlarged and is redder than normal. Dilated veins run across the capsular surface. The normal lobularity of the gland is accentuated.

160 and **161 The thyroid in 159 sliced transversly.** The cut surface has a mottled brown appearance.

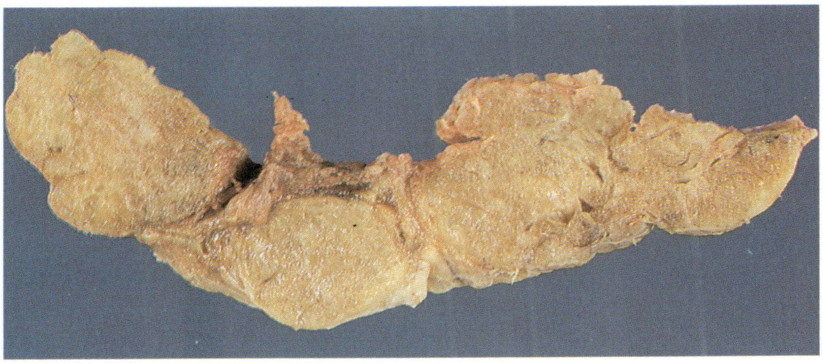

161

162 The thyroid gland from a patient with a multinodular goitre. In this case the nodularity involves the whole of the gland, but occasionally this is less well obvious and the isthmus is spared.

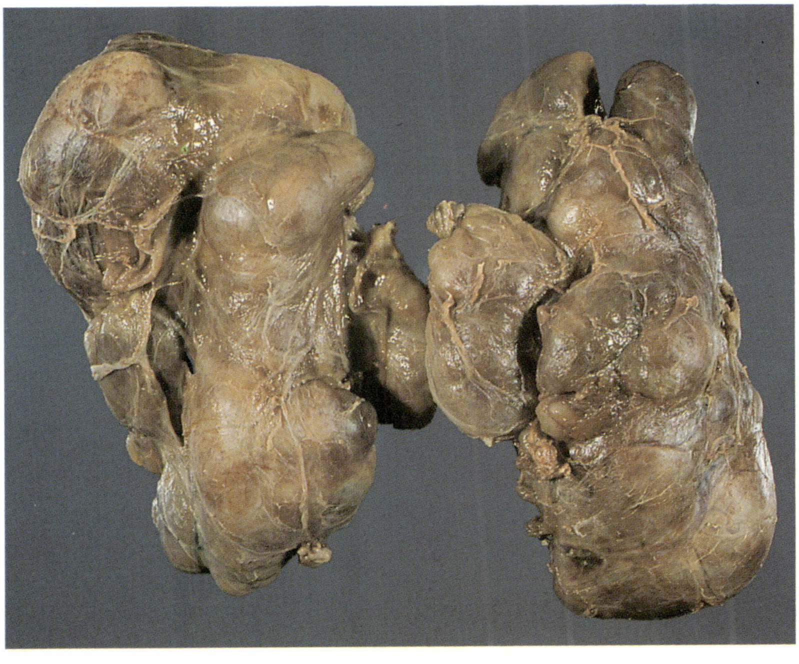

162

163

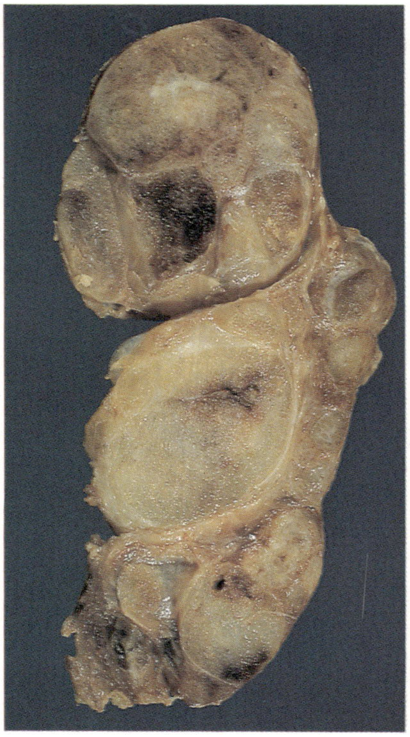

164

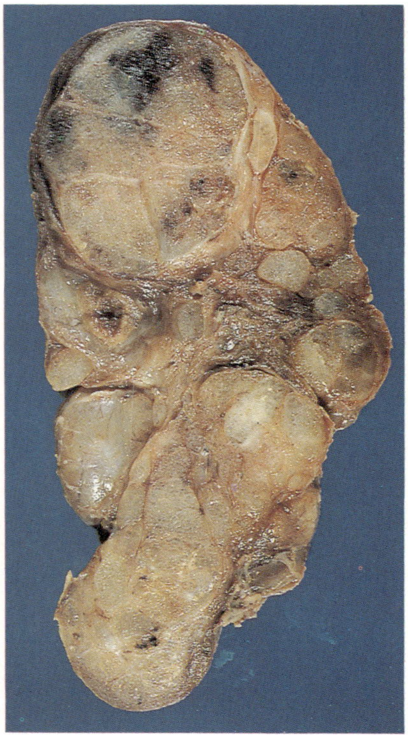

163 and 164 The thyroid in 162 sliced sagittally. Separated sections from both lobes show a typical variety in the size, colour and consistency of the nodules. In a case of thyrotoxicosis caused by a functioning nodule in a multinodular goitre, it is not possible to predict with confidence from the macroscopical or microscopical appearances which of the many nodules is responsible for the oversecretion.

165

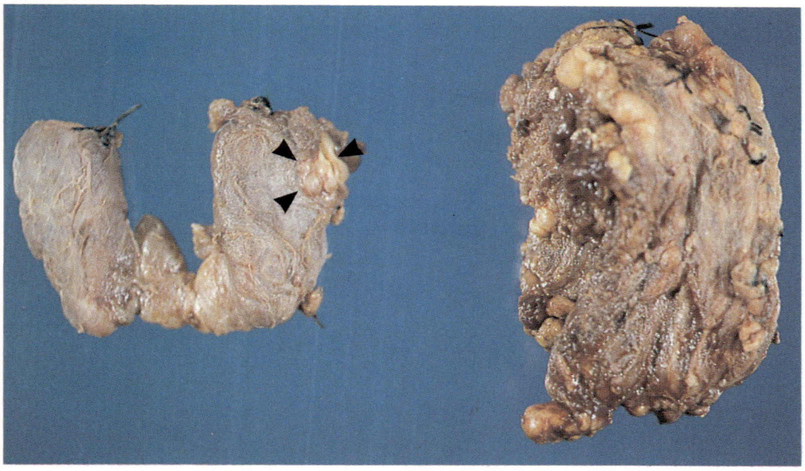

165 A total thyroidectomy and block dissection of the left side of the neck for carcinoma of the thyroid. The tumour (▶) involves the superolateral aspect of the left lobe.

166 A sagittal slice from 165 showing the lateral aspect of the thyroid gland. Part of the tumour has a distinct white fibrous capsule but this is deficient in the anterior aspect.

167 Transverse slices through 165, the block dissection of the neck. These show a mass of muscle, adipose and fibrous tissue enclosing nodules of white tumour tissue (some of which are replacing lymph nodes). On microscopic examination the tumour was found to be a papillary carcinoma of the thyroid.

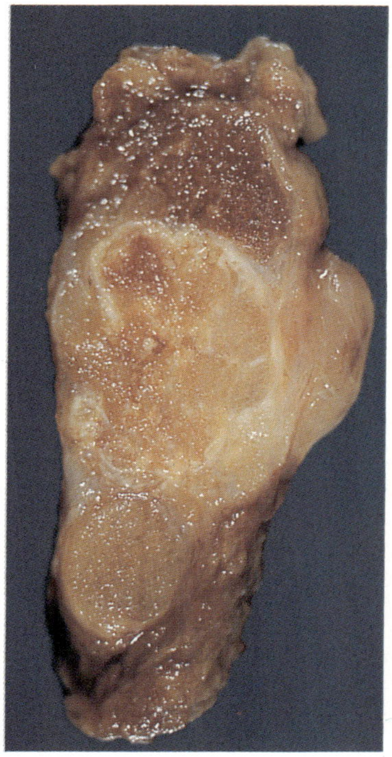

166

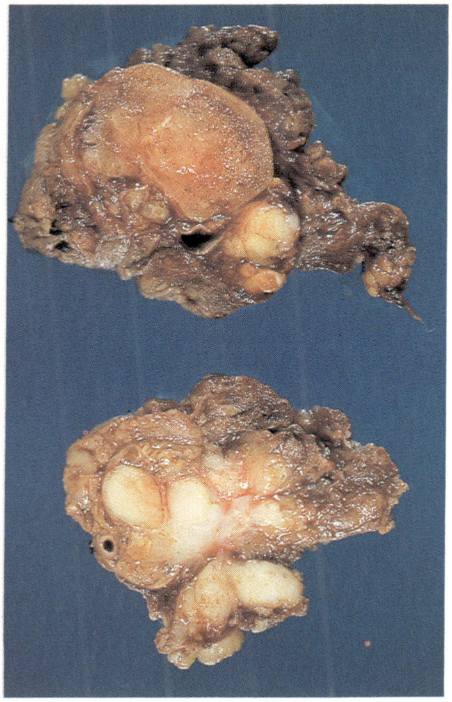

167

Parathyroid glands

Parathyroidectomy is performed for hyperparathyroidism. This is most commonly due to adenoma of the parathyroid glands but may be due to hyperplasia, which is either primary or secondary to hypocalcaemia, usually from chronic renal failure.

In most hospitals, the surgical treatment of hyperparathyroidism involves the excision of at least three and a half parathyroid glands (**168**). Because it is impossible to say with certainty whether an enlarged gland is hyperplastic or adenomatous without knowing the state of the other three, excision of a single gland is not indicated (**169**). The remaining half gland is left eutopically, or is sometimes transplanted subcutaneously or intramuscularly into the forearm, so that if subsequent hyperplasia or neoplasia occurs it can be more easily diagnosed and removed. The identification of parathyroid glands at operation with the naked eye is notoriously difficult, and imprint cytology or frozen sections are usually necessary to distinguish them from lymph nodes or small nodules of thyroid tissue. Very rarely, in surgically difficult cases where ectopic parathyroid glands are suspected (**170**), mediastinal adipose tissue may be received.

The weights and dimensions of the parathyroid glands should be recorded. The combined weight of four normal glands averages 120 mg. The number of glands can vary, and up to 12 have been recorded. It is of great importance that the sides and sites where the glands are taken are recorded, so that the report correlates with the operation notes and the surgeons can be directed to the correct area of the neck if there is a recurrence of hyperparathyroidism. The macroscopic appearances of a single gland are seldom helpful. Both hyperplastic and adenomatous glands are medium-brown or purple, and homogeneous on cut surface examination. The whole gland is blocked, unless it is large, in which case it is bisected and half is submitted.

Parathyroid glands: Macroscopical report	
Type of specimen	Side and site (upper or lower, right or left) of each gland (*very important*)
Measurements	Weight of each gland Size of each gland
Description	Short and simple description (e.g. 'A small ovoid brown fragment measuring . . . and weighing . . .')

168

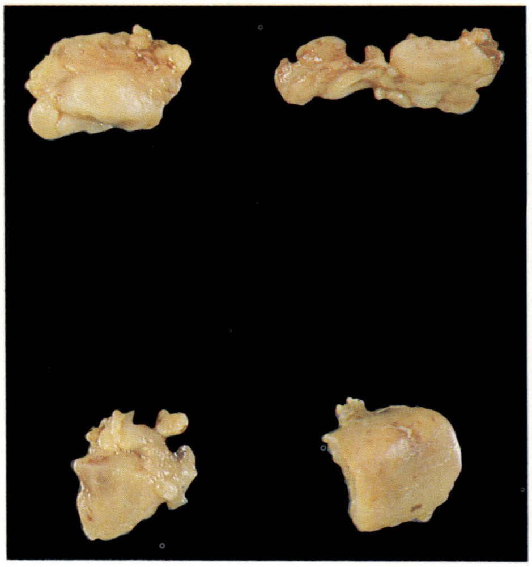

169

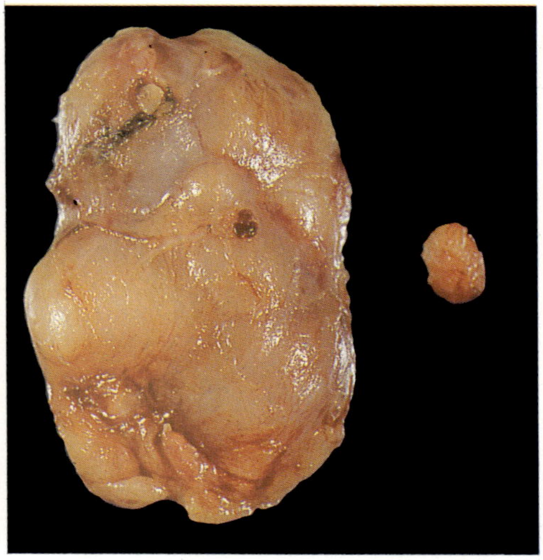

168 Four parathyroid glands from a patient with primary hyperparathyroidism. The combined weight of the glands was 230 mg (normal weight 120 mg).

169 A parathyroid adenoma weighing 1.6 g, together with a normal-sized gland from the same patient.

170

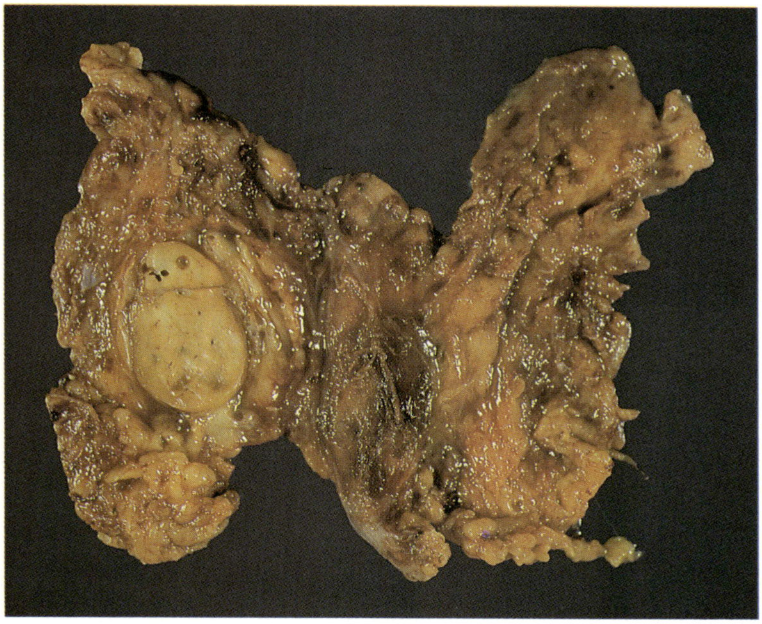

170 A mass of adipose tissue removed from the mediastinum of a patient with primary hyperparathyroidism. The discrete yellow mass is a parathyroid adenoma.

Endocrine pancreas

Islet cell neoplasms make up less than one per cent of pancreatic tumours. They are more frequent in the tail and body of the pancreas, corresponding to the greater concentration of islets in these sites, and may be multiple (**171a**). The tissue received is therefore usually a partial (distal) pancreatectomy specimen with or without a splenectomy specimen. If the spleen is present, it should be removed and treated as described on p 102. Endocrine tumours form rounded nodules with cut surfaces which show uniform pink or white tissue. Longstanding tumours may be firm because of increasing amounts of fibrosis.

The excision margin of the pancreas should be marked with India ink, and removed for blocks before further dissection. The specimen should then be sectioned at 1 cm intervals transversely across the pancreatic duct. Blocks are taken to illustrate the position of the tumour(s) in relation to the pancreatic duct, the capsule and the peripancreatic tissues, if present. Where there are multiple tumours, blocks should be taken from each and labelled separately (**171b**).

Endocrine pancreas: Macroscopical report

Type of specimen	Needle core of tissue, irregular tissue fragment, partial pancreatectomy (For Whipple's operation, see p 36)
Measurements	Size and weight
Description	
Outer surface	Colour (haemorrhages, grey tissue necrosis, yellow fat necrosis); contour (distortion by tumour, scarring); consistency (soft, firm, focally calcified)
Focal lesions	Number; sizes and sites of tumour nodules; cut surface appearance (as above: colour; consistency)
Rest of gland	Colour; consistency; appearance of main duct
Other tissues	Spleen; lymph nodes

Example 171

The specimen consists of a distal pancreatectomy measuring 9.5 × 4.3 × 0.8 cm. At the proximal end there is a soft, circumscribed, nodular tumour mass measuring 3.1 cm in diameter, which appears to extend to the excision margin. A second tumour mass which has an ill-defined edge and measures 2.6 cm in diameter is present in the distal part of the specimen. Just medial to this, below the superior surface, there is a third tumour, 1.5 cm in diameter.

The cut surface of each tumour shows soft pink and purple tissue with tiny areas of haemorrhage. The pancreatic tissue around the tumours has the normal lobulated brown appearance, but in the centre of the specimen there is a thin-walled cyst 1.8 cm in diameter containing clear fluid. This does not appear to be involved by tumour. No lymph nodes are found in the specimen.

Blocks

A pancreatic resection margin × 2
B proximal tumour mass × 2
C distal tumour mass × 1
D central tumour mass × 1
E cyst wall × 1
F uninvolved pancreas × 1

171a

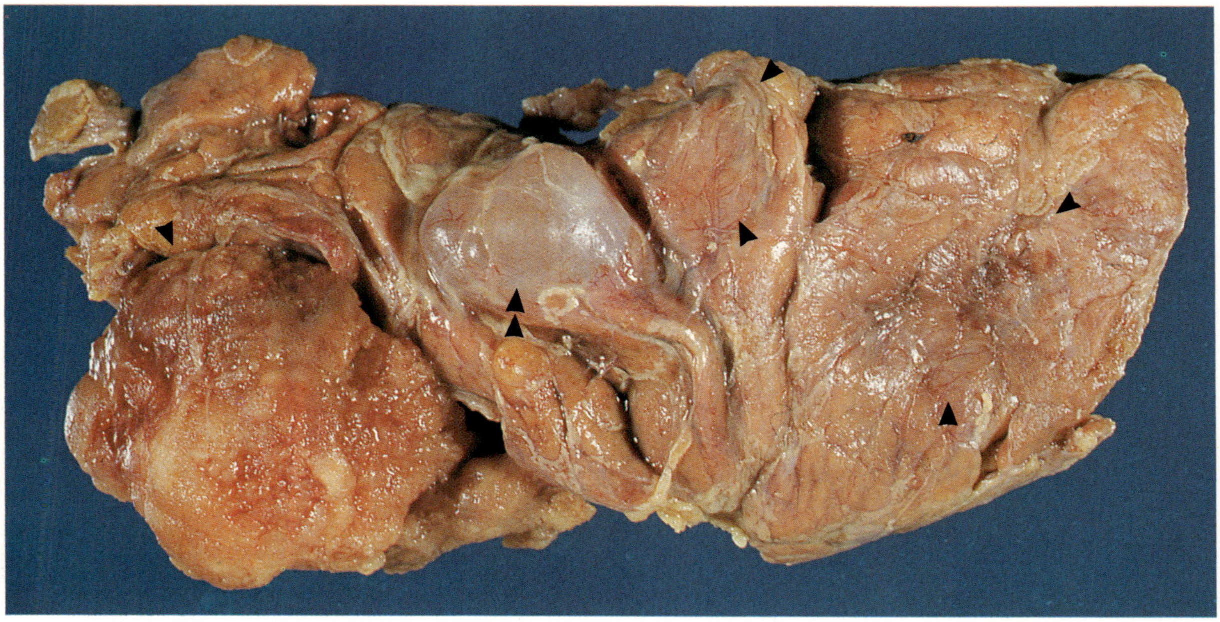

171a The external surface and excision margin of a distal pancreatectomy specimen performed for multiple islet cell tumours (▶). A thin-walled cyst is also present (▶▶).

171b

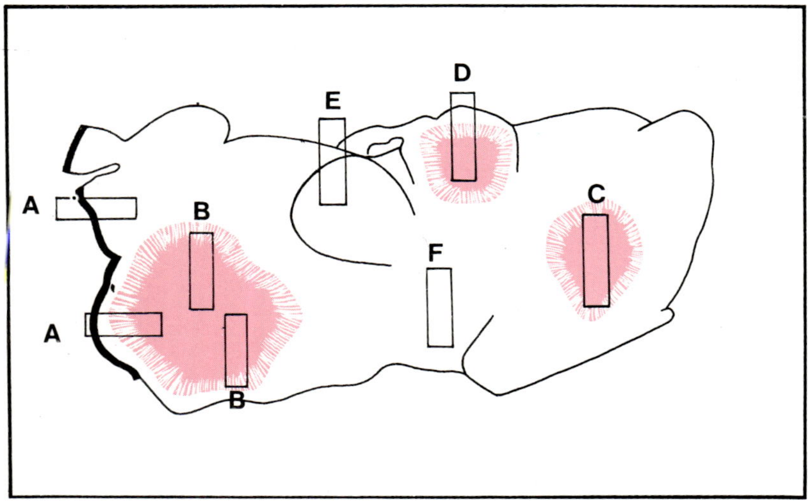

171b Blocks from a partial pancreatectomy for endocrine disease. If a tumour is too large to include central and peripheral parts in one block, more than one block should be taken. If tumours are multiple, at least one block from each should be taken. Pancreatic excision margin (**A**); proximal tumour mass (**B**); distal tumour mass (**C**); central tumour mass (**D**); other focal lesions such as cyst wall (**E**); uninvolved pancreas (**F**).

CHAPTER 11
HEAD AND NECK

Ear, nose, oral cavity and larynx

Small specimens

Mucosal biopsies may be taken for the diagnosis of inflammation and neoplasia of the mastoid antrum, vestibule, nasal spaces and sinuses, post nasal space, mouth, pharynx and larynx. The number and sites should be specified. The description, as for mucosal biopsies elsewhere, is usually very short ('A small fragment of pink tissue measuring . . .') and the specimen is embedded whole. If a mucosal surface can be identified, the tissue should be embedded so that it is sectioned at right angles to the epithelium; orientation, however, is often impossible.

Inflammatory nasal polyps are the most common larger specimens (**172**). These are translucent, gelatinous rounded masses ranging from about 0.5 to 3 cm in diameter. Examination of the cut surface shows a homogenous pink or grey colour. Small cystic areas may be present, and focal collections of inflammatory cells appear as dense white patches. Areas of calcification or fragments of bone are common in nasal polypectomy specimens and if present the tissue should be decalcified. Half of each polyp should be blocked.

A nasal polyp composed of firm, opaque, dense pink or white tissue may be neoplastic rather than inflammatory. Inverted squamous cell papilloma (Ringert's tumour, Schneiderian papilloma, transitional cell papilloma) has a tendency to local recurrence, and after repeated recurrence may become fully malignant as a metastasizing squamous cell carcinoma.

Cysts removed from the lip, gingiva or tongue range in size from tiny fragments of tissue to recognizable cystic structures some centimetres in diameter. Small cysts may be embedded whole; larger ones may be bisected or cut into parallel slices.

Adenoids and tonsils may be removed because of chronic inflammation or neoplasia. They consist of irregular pink or purple masses of soft tissue, over which a mucosal covering may be identifiable. Parallel cuts are made through larger fragments and blocks selected from the mucosa, dense white areas and other focal lesions. In cases of neoplasia, marking of the excision margins is seldom necessary as the operation is performed to provide tissue for diagnosis rather than as a curative procedure.

Pharyngeal pouches may be excised, and

Small specimens, ear, nose and oral cavity: Macroscopical report	
Site	Sites of biopsies must be recorded as precisely as possible
Type of specimen	Tissue fragment, mucosal biopsy, cyst, polyp(s), mass of tissue partly covered by mucosa
Measurements	Number and sizes of the specimens in three planes, or maximum dimension if very small
Description	Colour Surface appearance (smooth, glistening, granular, papillary, rounded, irregular, ovoid) Consistency (soft, rubbery, watery, friable) Cut surface (gelatinous, haemorrhagic, dense and solid, focal yellow areas)

consist of false diverticula of mucosa, usually herniated through the inferior constrictor muscle in the neck. They should be opened longitudinally (**173**) and the presence of mucosal abnormality (ulcer, tumour) noted.

Laryngectomy specimens

Laryngectomy is performed for carcinoma of the larynx, and rarely for other laryngeal or pharyngeal neoplasms. The specimen includes the lower pharynx, epiglottis, larynx and upper trachea, and surrounding structures such as the thyroid and hyoid bone, and overlying skin if involved by tumour (**174, 175**).

It is necessary to determine the tumour type that is present, its differentiation and how far it has spread. The first two are usually easy, but the last can be extremely difficult because of the complicated topography of the area. The principal features which must be addressed in the macroscopic report are the sites of origin and involvement by tumour (whether supraglottic, glottic, transglottic or infraglottic), and whether the surgical excision lines have been reached.

There are several methods described for dissection of a laryngectomy specimen. Some involve sagittal sectioning of the specimen, which produces very large blocks. This method defines the position of a tumour in relation to the vocal cords, epiglottis and trachea. Transverse sections taken close together and labelled in sequence have also been advocated.

One method currently in use at the Institute of Laryngology and Otology, London, involves fixing the entire specimen in 10 per cent buffered formalin for at least 48 hours. It is then opened with a vertical cut through the posterior surface (**175**) and the gross appearances are recorded. The hyoid bone is removed, decalcified and submitted for histology. The specimen is then sequentially sliced transversely at 4 mm intervals using a commercial meat-slicing machine. Alternatively, the entire specimen can be decalcified and cut with a long-bladed knife. These methods display the tumour and surrounding soft tissues (**176**). The slices should be numbered or lettered sequentially and photographed, to facilitate the orientation of the subsequent histological sections and the identification of the excision margins. The slices can be divided into blocks of appropriate size and decalcified if necessary before processing. They may be outlined on the photographs so that correlation with the microscopical appearances is possible. Depending on the extent of involvement by tumour, it may not be necessary to embed the entire larynx, and selected slices could be used for blocks (**176**).

Larynx: Macroscopical report

Type of specimen	Laryngectomy specimen with cervical lymph nodes, and overlying thyroid gland, hyoid bone, anterior strap muscles and skin
Measurements	Length of specimen, diameter of larynx, pharynx and upper trachea Dimensions of attached tissues
Description	
Tumour	Sites (involvement of named parts of specimen—true cords, hyoid bone, trachea, false cords, epiglottis, etc.); bilaterality of tumour Size of tumour Colour; consistency; contour (papillary, ulcerated, infiltrative) Involvement of extralaryngeal structures and excision margins
Rest of larynx	Appearance of non-neoplastic mucosa over cords, etc.
Other tissues	Thyroid, parathyroids, skin, lymph nodes, muscles, etc.

Example 174-176

The specimen consists of a total laryngectomy with an attached thyroid gland and an overlying rectangular portion of skin and subcutis. It measures 9.1 cm from epiglottis to tracheal resection margin and the larynx is 4.9 cm in greatest diameter. The skin measures 7 × 5.5 cm and includes a tracheostomy site.

Around the tracheostomy on the anterior laryngeal mucosa, there is a soft, haemorrhagic, partially ulcerated mass measuring 3.1 cm in diameter. This extends from the true vocal cords to 1 cm from the tracheal resection margin. The cut section shows that the tumour has invaded the hyoid bone and thyroid cartilage to involve the overlying skin. There is a separate red tumour nodule, 1.1 cm in diameter, within the paratracheal soft tissues on the left side. The thyroid gland contains a firm white nodule 1.2 cm in diameter. The consistency and colour of the nodule are different from the laryngeal tumour. Apart from this nodule, the thyroid appears normal. No parathyroid glands or lymph nodes are found in the specimen.

Blocks

A embedded in 4 pieces
B-G each embedded in 3 pieces
H, J both embedded in 2 pieces

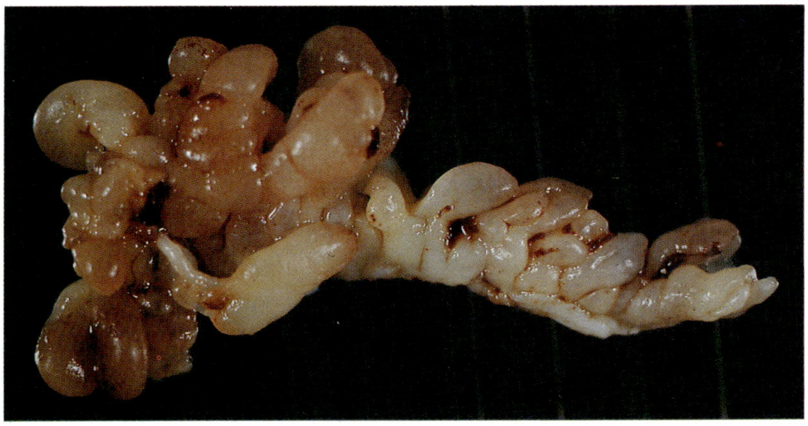

172

172 A strip of nasal mucosa bearing several inflammatory nasal polyps with a typical lobulated pink and red gelatinous appearance.

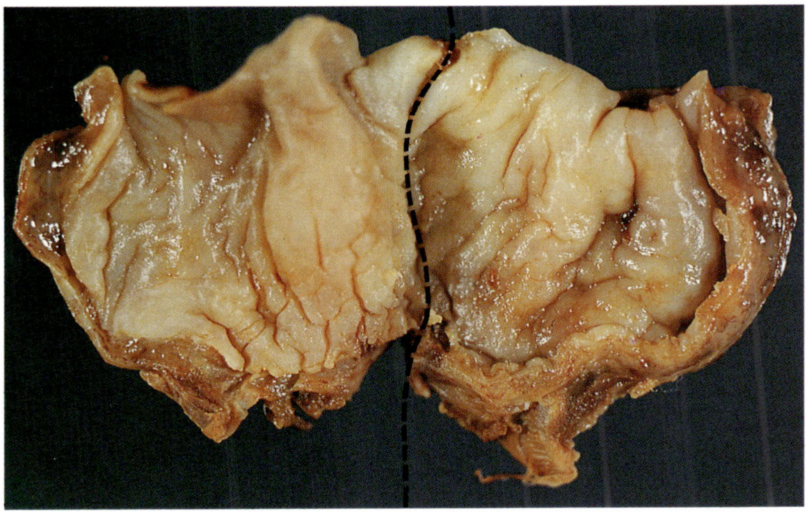

173

173 A false diverticulum of the pharynx. The specimen has been bisected longitudinally (the hinge is indicated by a broken line). The mouth of the diverticulum is at the top and there is a small ulcer on its left lateral wall with oedema of the adjacent mucosa.

174

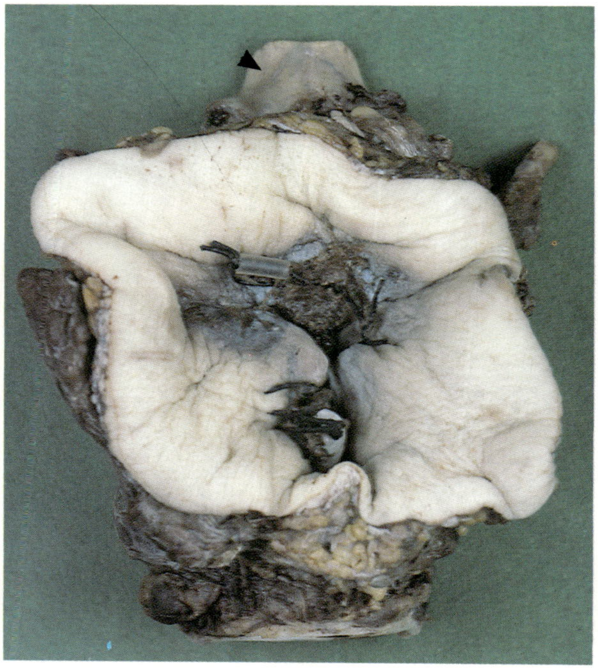

175

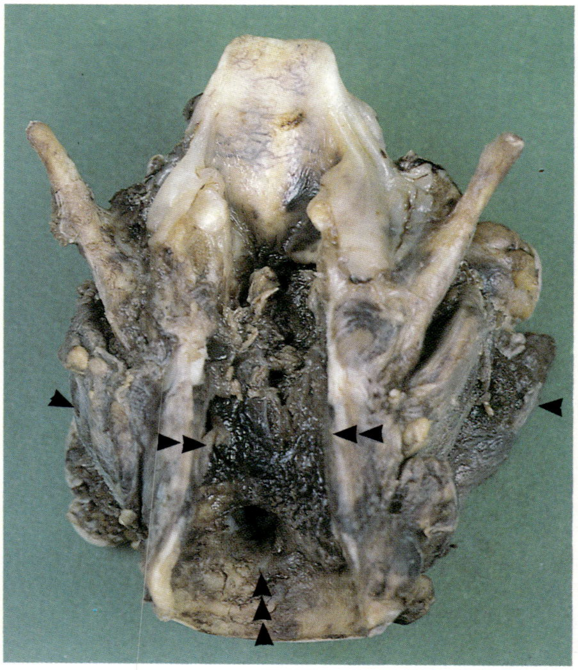

174 An extended laryngectomy specimen, anterior view. The skin of the anterior aspect of the neck has been excised because of involvement by a laryngeal neoplasm. The dark-blue discoloration is methylene blue used at the operation. It delineates the area of skin invaded by tumour. Below this is a tracheostomy opening. The anterior surface of the epiglottis can be seen at the top of the specimen (▶).

175 Specimen 174 opened through the posterior aspect. The structures that can be identified are, from the top: the epiglottis (top centre); the twin horns of the hyoid bone (top left and right); the thyroid gland (▶); the area of the vocal cords replaced by tumour (▶▶); and the tracheostomy site (▶▶▶).

176

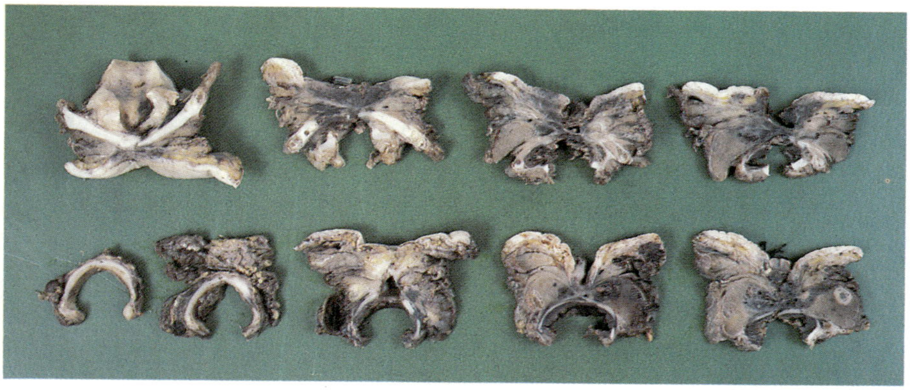

176 Specimen 174 after transverse sectioning. The tissue slices have been laid out in sequence for further fixation if necessary and decalcification. The first slice has been inverted to show the upper resection margin. This tumour was found microscopically to be an angiosarcoma.

Salivary glands

Small biopsies are rarely taken from major salivary glands. The whole or a large part of a gland may be excised for the treatment of chronic inflammation (with or without sialolithiasis) and salivary gland tumours (177).

Dissection of specimen

The specimen is generally fixed whole and dissected after fixation. When calculi are suspected, specimen radiography should be performed if possible. The surgical excision margins of a specimen should be carefully identified and marked with India ink. This is particularly important for salivary gland tumours, which may appear circumscribed but under the microscope may be seen to extend into the surrounding connective tissues for some distance from the parent mass.

The specimen is measured and the outer aspect described. Parallel slices are cut through the tissue as thinly as possible without fragmentation of the specimen (177). The cut surface can then be examined. Tumours and areas of heterogeneity are described and the presence of calculi noted. Calculi should be removed if possible. If not, the whole specimen should be decalcified before processing.

A search should be made for nerve trunks and other cord-like structures on the surface of the specimen or running through it. In the parotid gland, facial nerve branches may be involved by tumour.

Blocks should be taken from areas of tumour and other focal lesions, and from adjacent tissues and resection margins to demonstrate the extent of involvement. When the cut surface is heterogeneous, all of the different areas should be sampled.

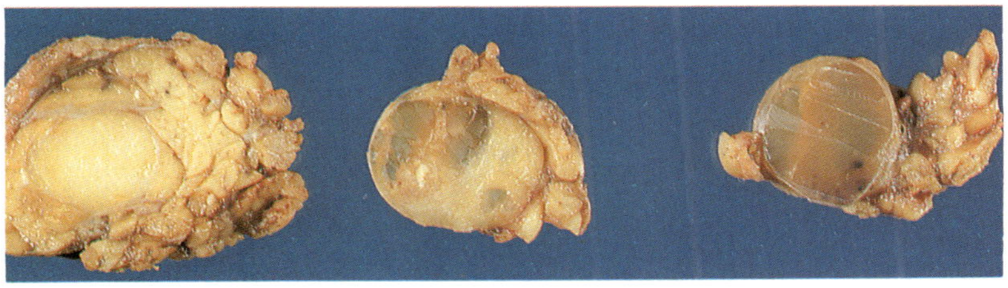

177

177 **Sequential slices through a parotid tumour** which was found microscopically to be a monomorphic adenoma. The tumour is well circumscribed and composed partly of solid white tissue and partly of gelatinous material within cystic spaces. The surrounding salivary tissue shows no macroscopic abnormality.

Salivary glands: Macroscopical report	
Type of specimen	Parotidectomy, sialadenectomy, irregular mass of tissue
Measurements	Maximum dimensions in three planes
Description	
Outer surface	Colour; texture (rough, glistening, translucent); contour (rounded, irregular, ill-defined); attached connective tissues (adipose tissue, muscle, bone)
Cut surface	*Focal lesions* Size; colour (uniform pink, variegated yellow, grey and white); contour (well-defined, irregular, indistinct); consistency (mucoid, firm, rubbery, hard); relation to surrounding tissues and excision margin *Rest of gland* Colour; uniformity (dilated ducts, haemorrhage, cysts); presence of calculi, and their number, sizes and sites; presence of nerve trunks or other cords of tissue

CHAPTER 12

OSTEOARTICULAR SYSTEM AND SOFT TISSUES

Bone and cartilage

Small specimens

Trephine needle biopsies of bone may be taken to investigate osteolytic or sclerotic lesions where there is suspicion of metastatic tumour deposits; or they may be taken for the diagnosis of metabolic bone disease or for the diagnosis of haematological disorders. If metabolic bone disease is suspected, buffered formalin at pH 7 should be used as a fixative to preserve the mineralization of the bone. Rarely, trephine biopsies may be taken for the diagnosis of primary bone tumours. Descriptions of such biopsies are usually brief, for example, 'A needle core of bony tissue . . . cm in length'.

Open biopsy specimens from the iliac crest provide larger and therefore more representative samples for quantitation of osteoid and mineralized bone for the diagnosis of metabolic bone disease. Resin embedding and a motorized microtome with a hardened blade are necessary to produce undecalcified sections.

Fragments may be curetted from bone tumours or cases of osteomyelitis. If infection is suspected and unfixed tissue is available, a sample should be sent for microbiological examination – this can be returned and processed for histology after inoculation of culture media.

Bony fragments need decalcifying and thereafter can usually be embedded whole; if not, larger pieces should be cut after decalcification to minimize fragmentation. Small particles of bone are often sent with fibrocartilage resected for the treatment of prolapsed intervertebral disc; if the fragments feel hard, they should be decalcified before processing. The aggregate volume of the tissue should be measured and most or all of the specimen should be embedded.

Large specimens

Large specimens range from femoral heads (see below) and local resections of benign tumours to parts of long bones and entire limbs removed for malignancy, arterial disease or trauma.

Amputation specimens are uncommon and can be complicated to dissect. Advice should be sought from experienced colleagues if at all possible.

Dissection of specimen

The approach to dissection will depend upon the reason for resection.

Resections for malignant disease

In some parts of the USA, necropsy permission must be obtained before an amputation specimen is dissected. If possible,

Bone biopsy: Macroscopical report	
Type of specimen	Needle core of bone, curettings, irregular bony fragment, wedge of bone
Measurements	Length, maximum dimensions or aggregate volume
Description	Colour Consistency (bony, cartilaginous, fibrous)

the pathologist dealing with a bone, digit or limb removed for malignant disease should discuss the pre-operative radiographs with the clinicians or radiologists before dissection. This saves time by helping to establish whether a tumour is within, attached to or adjacent to the bone, whether there is fracture with callus formation and whether the lesion is predominantly cystic or solid. The radiographs also indicate sites where blocks should be taken for radiological interest, and cortical thickening in Paget's disease can be easily seen.

In disarticulations and other large specimens for primary bone tumours and soft tissue tumours, it is important that the macroscopic appearances are fully recorded. Photography is very useful for recording the appearances of an amputated limb and can save pages of written description. Photographs should be taken of the entire specimen, of the external aspect of the area in which the pathology is sited, and of the bones and joints after dissection.

The pathologist should determine:

- the site of origin of a tumour (e.g. medullary, subperiosteally, in the epiphysis or metaphysis).
- the gross appearance and local extent of the tumour.
- whether joint spaces are involved.
- the extent of spread along the medullary cavity, and subperiosteal extension.
- the relation to vessels and nerves.
- the proximity to excision lines.

Handling for a limb removed for malignancy starts with the measurement of the specimen. The first aspects to be dissected are the resection ends of the neurovascular bundle and the soft tissues if these might be involved. Next, the skin and soft tissues away from the tumour are removed (**178a, 179**) if these are present. A search should be made for lymph nodes, especially in antecubital and popliteal fossae. If surgery has produced a cut end of bone rather than a disarticulation, a transverse block of the resection end should be taken at this stage. The bone is then cut with a band saw.

For sarcomas arising in the medulla or growing circumferentially around the shaft of a bone, longitudinal sectioning of the bone is

Resections for malignant disease: Macroscopical report	
Types of specimen	Below or above knee/elbow amputation, forequarter or hindquarter amputation, digit, length of femur or tibia, hemimandibulectomy, etc.
Measurements of specimen	The length of the bone or limb and of its component parts (e.g. length from excision end to knee, knee to heel, heel to end of great toe) Maximum circumference of thigh, leg, etc. Maximum circumference of limb at site of tumour before dissection
Description	Site of origin of the tumour (medulla, below the periosteum, in the epiphysis, metaphysis or diaphysis) Size (maximum dimensions in three planes) Distance of tumour from epiphyseal plate and excision end of bone (this may need adjusting after histological sections have been examined, as spread may be more extensive than can be appreciated macroscopically) Extent of subperiosteal spread, if present Extent of local extension into surrounding tissues; relation of tumour with vessels and nerves Contour; colour; consistency of the tumour Number, sites and appearance of lymph nodes in the specimen Other pathology present in the specimen (skin lesions, previous biopsy sites) Appearance of joints and bones away from the tumour

usually best (**180a**). When the tumour arises eccentrically, as is often the case with soft tissue tumours, the bone can be cut transversely with a band saw at 1-2 cm intervals. This latter method is also used with flat or irregularly-shaped bones (**181, 182, 183**). If soft tissues are present, the cuts are then extended almost through the specimen with a long-bladed knife to produce either a 'book' dissection (as for breast and spleen) or a series of separate cross sections which should be kept in sequence.

Careful labelling of the sites from which the blocks are obtained is important, and is best done on a photograph. Extensive sampling of a tumour, including any soft, fibrous, chondroid, cystic or haemorrhagic areas, is essential. Blocks from peripheral lobules of neoplastic tissue in tumours such as chrondrosarcoma and osteosarcoma are more rewarding than blocks from the centre of these tumours, where maturation of the neoplastic cells may make diagnosis more difficult. In osteosarcoma, tissue from Codman's angle, between the lifted periosteum and cortical bone, is often unrewarding and may show only reactive non-neoplastic bone. Blocks are also taken from the surrounding bone, and from the overlying skin, lymph nodes and other tissues if present (**178b, 180b**).

Example 178-180

The specimen is an amputated distal end of femur measuring 16.4 cm in length. There is an attached ellipse of pale skin 8 cm long and 1.1 cm in maximum width. This contains a healing surgical scar compatible with the site of the previous biopsy. Soft tissue is also attached to the posterior surface of the bone in the distal third, over a length of 6 cm.

Sagittal slicing of the specimen shows a firm white tumour mass projecting from the posterior surface of the metaphysis, which is arising subperiosteally. The original cortical bone at the distal posterior surface of the metaphysis has disappeared, and the tumour extends through the overlying periosteum into the adjacent fibrous tissue, but does not appear macroscopically to penetrate the medullary cavity to any extent. The tumour measures 6.2 cm in length and 1.3 cm in maximum thickness, and lies 8.1 cm from the femoral excision margin.

The bone away from the tumour appears normal, and there is no abnormality present in the articular cartilage or muscles. No lymph nodes are found in the popliteal aspect of the specimen, and no neurovascular bundle has been excised in this case.

Blocks

- A skin and subcutaneous tissue overlying tumour × 2
- B muscle adjacent to tumour × 2
- C excision end of femur × 2
- D tumour × 3
- E medullary bone deep to tumour × 1
- F articular cartilage adjacent to tumour × 1
- G medullary bone away from tumour × 1

Resections for ischaemia and trauma

The specimen should be measured and carefully examined externally. In ischaemic limbs or digits longitudinal incisions should then be made along the lines of the neurovascular bundles to identify the major arteries and veins (**184, 185, 186**). These can either be opened longitudinally with fine scissors or cut transversely along their lengths to look for atheroma, thrombus and other pathology. Blocks are taken from representative areas of diseased vessels, ischaemic soft tissues and areas of gangrene. Soft tissue resection margins should be taken to assess viability, but it is not usually necessary to examine blocks of bone.

Traumatized limbs or digits should be extensively photographed and X-rayed if there is any question of medicolegal involvement. A full description of the state of the tissues and an assessment of the possible causative agent (e.g. blunt trauma, stabbing, crushing, burning) should be recorded. Microscopic examination is seldom of great value but blocks should be taken from the resection line to see whether the tissue appears viable. The soft tissues are then removed and blocks taken from fractures to try to assess the duration of healing and to exclude the possibility of pathological fracture.

Resections for ischaemia and trauma: Macroscopical report	
Types of specimen	Below or above knee/elbow amputation, foot, digit, etc.
Measurements	The length of the limb and of its component parts (e.g. length from excision end to knee, knee to heel, heel to end of great toe) Maximum circumference of thigh, leg, etc.
Description	
Lesions	Types (ulcers, areas of discoloration, bruising, types of wound, surgical incisions, scars, gangrene) Number and size of lesions, and extent of involvement of the limb
Rest of specimen	State of the skin: colour; texture (thin, hairless, ulcerated); identifying marks (tattoos, old scars, etc) Appearance of the arteries and veins after dissection: extent of atheroma, thrombosis; extent of obliteration of lumen Appearance of other tissues, such as muscles, bones, joints

Lesions of joints and para-articular tissues

Small cysts and biopsies from or adjacent to joints can usually be described briefly, measured, and embedded whole. With larger cysts (**187**) a short macroscopical report is given, and representative portions of the wall should be taken. If gout is suspected in a joint, biopsies should be fixed in alcohol rather than formalin. This will preserve the water-soluble urate crystals, allowing a more positive diagnosis.

Femoral heads with osteoarthrosis should be examined, measured and described. Adherent joint capsule should be removed, and the bone then cut into slices with a band saw through the articular surface in line with the femoral neck (**188, 189**). Blocks can be taken from the slices of bone after decalcification.

Femoral heads: Macroscopical report	
Measurements	Diameter of head, maximum thickness of articular cartilage, length of femoral neck
Description	
Articular surface	Smooth and glistening, roughened, fibrillation of cartilage, eburnation of bone surface, osteophyte formation, granulation tissue formation (pannus)
Cut surface	Bone cysts, subarticular haemorrhage, fibrosis, fracture within specimen
Attached soft tissues	Overgrowth of synovium with villus formation, congestion and oedema, brown discoloration, capsular fibrosis

Example 188-189

The specimen is a head of femur measuring 5.5 cm in diameter, with 0.8 cm of attached femoral neck. The articular surface shows extensive loss of cartilage with severe eburnation and haemorrhagic discoloration of the bone. Cut sections show irregular cystic spaces measuring up to 1 cm in maximum dimension in the subchondral bone. There is no evidence of Paget's disease of bone, tumour or fracture callus.

Blocks × 3

178a

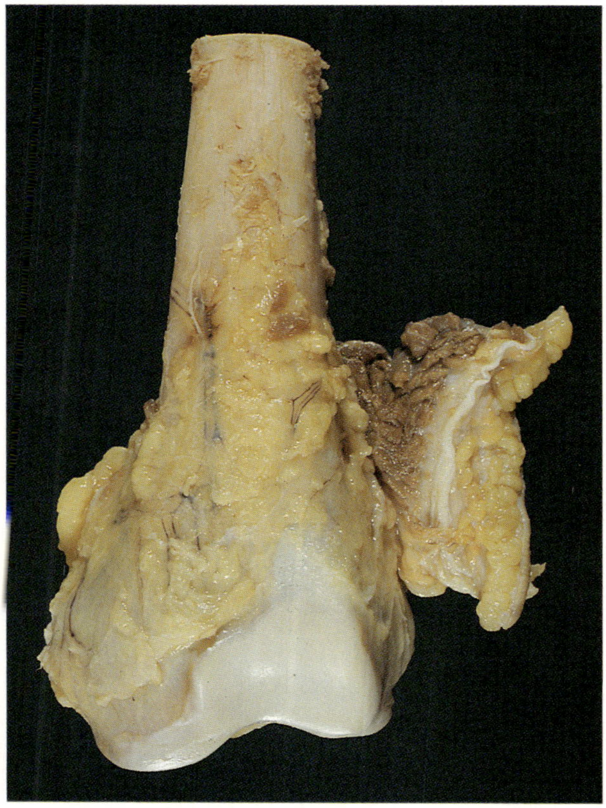

179

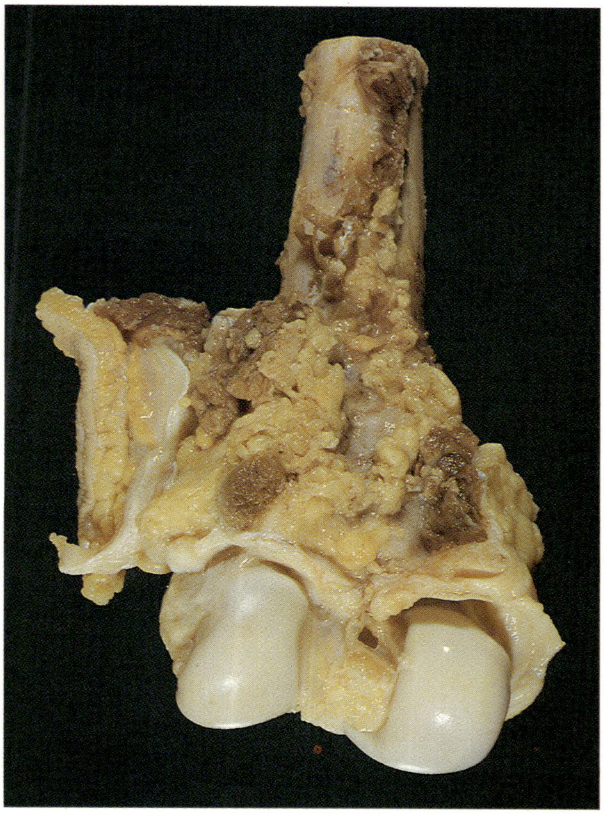

178a and 179 The distal third of the femur amputated for parosteal osteosarcoma (a mass of muscle and skin overlying the tumour was also excised). The tumour is obscured by the soft tissues in these views. (The patient was given a prosthetic lower femur and knee joint.)

178b Blocks taken from an amputation specimen with bone or cartilage tumour, Part 1 (for Part 2, see **180b**): skin and subcutaneous tissue overlying tumour (**A**); muscle adjacent to tumour (**B**).

178b

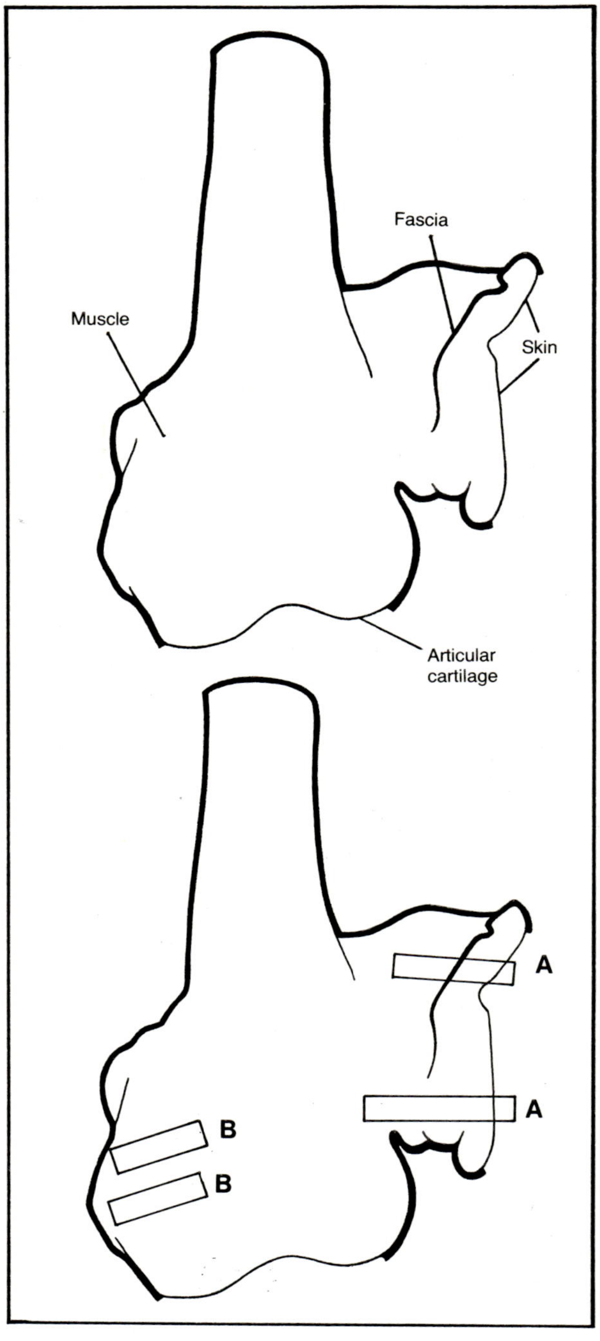

180a A sagittal, longitudinal section of the femur in 178 and 179 showing the tumour mass projecting from the posterior surface of the metaphysis.

180b Blocks taken from an amputation specimen with bone or cartilage tumour, Part 2: excision end of femur (**C**), tumour (**D**), medullary bone adjacent to tumour (**E**); articular cartilage (**F**); medullary bone away from tumour (**G**).

180a

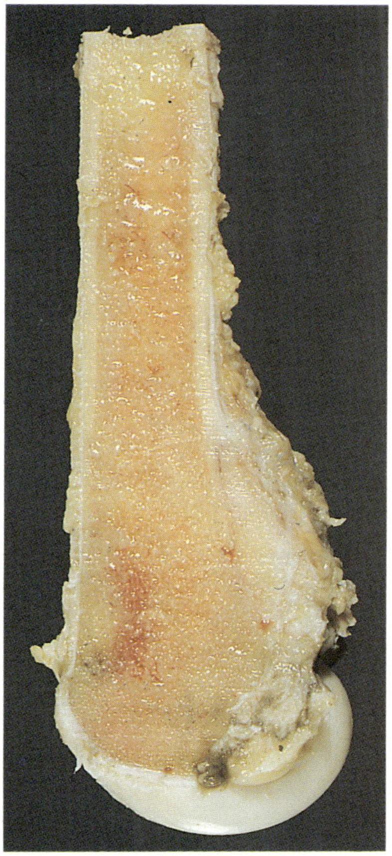

180b

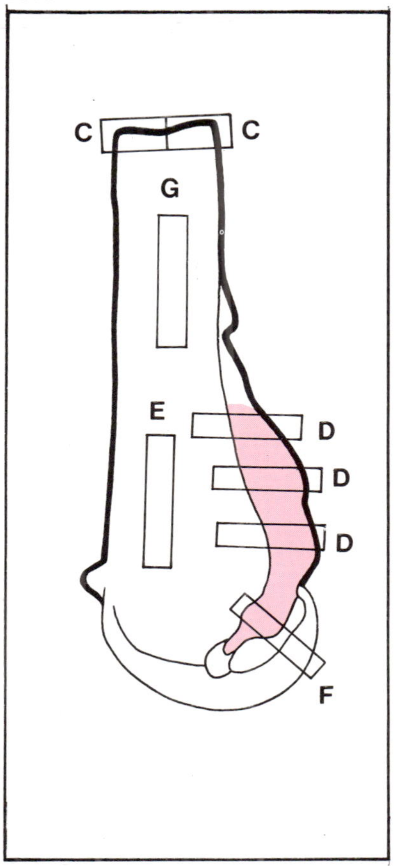

181

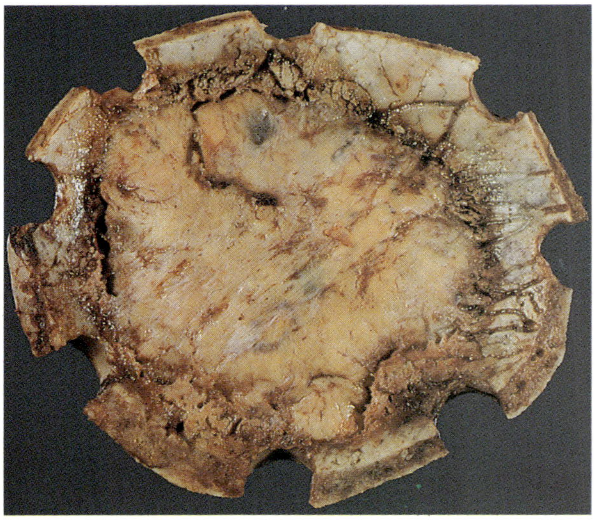

182

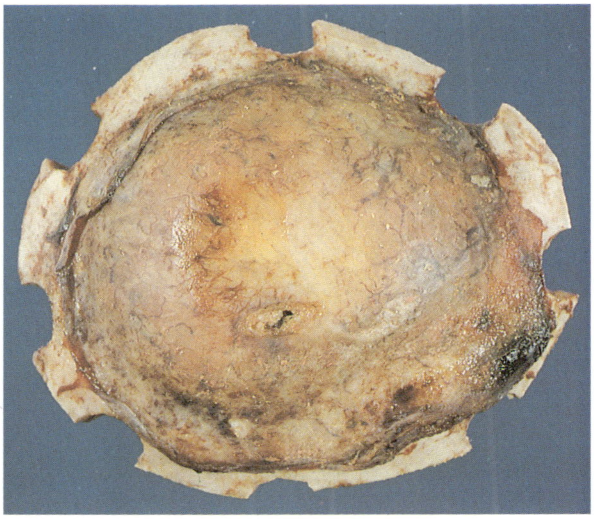

181 and 182 A metastatic tumour deposit in the skull from a primary follicular carcinoma of the thyroid (inner aspect **181**, outer aspect **182**). The periosteum on the outer surface is intact; the dura over the inner surface was stripped and not excised.

183

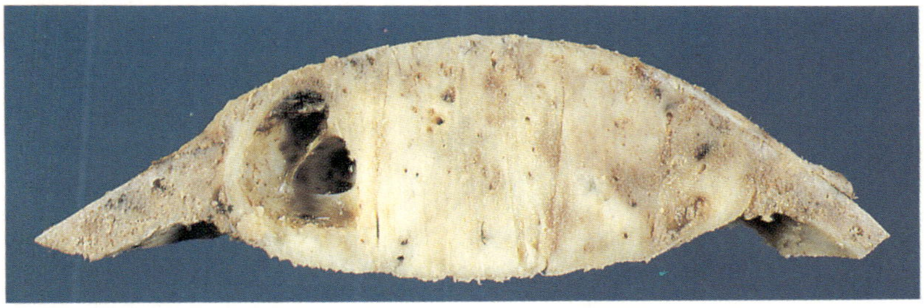

183 A section of 181, 182, the skull containing a metastatic carcinoma. The tumour expands the tables of the skull and the cut surface is mostly solid and composed of pink and grey tissue. Cyst formation has occurred in one place.

184

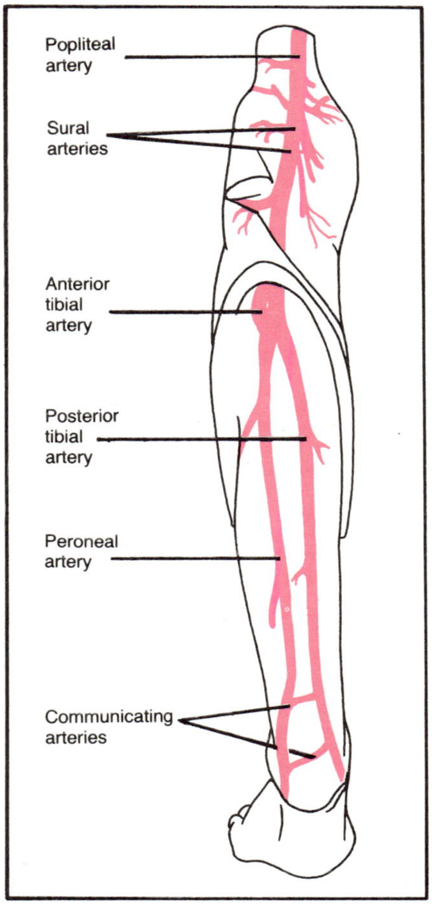

185

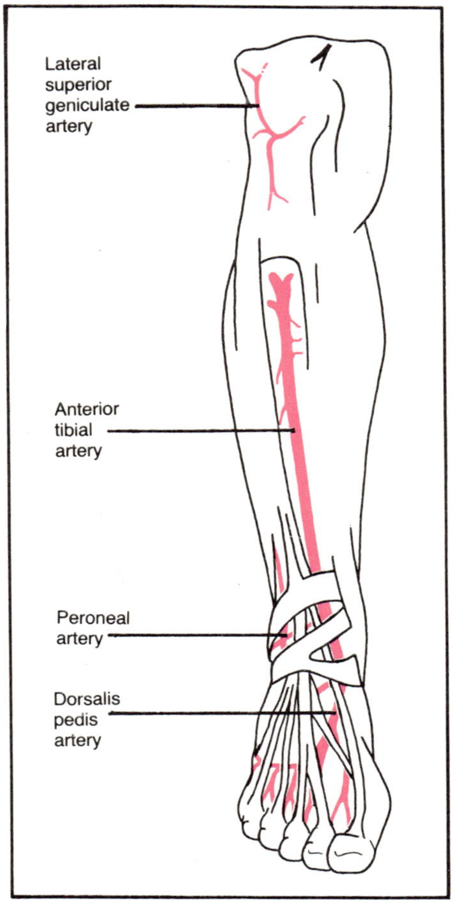

186

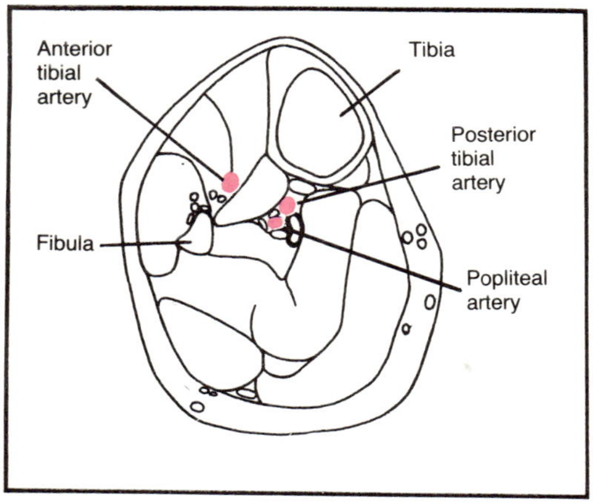

184, 185 and **186 Blood supplies to the lower limbs.**

187 A prepatellar bursa. The specimen consists of sheets of glistening homogeneous white tissue. A small amount of adipose tissue is adherent to the surface.

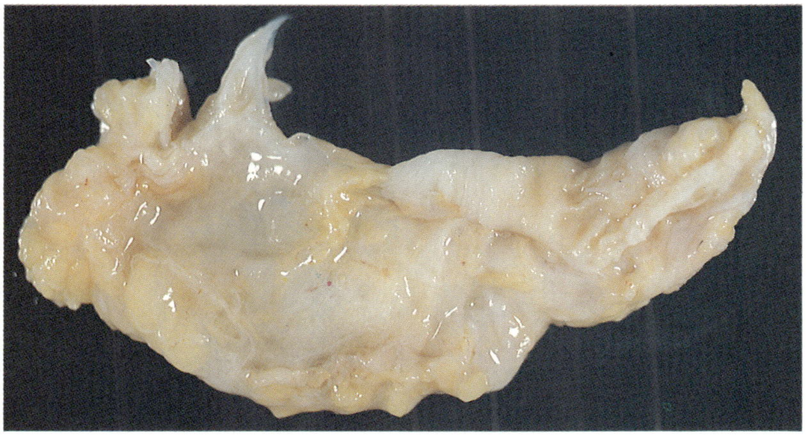

187

88

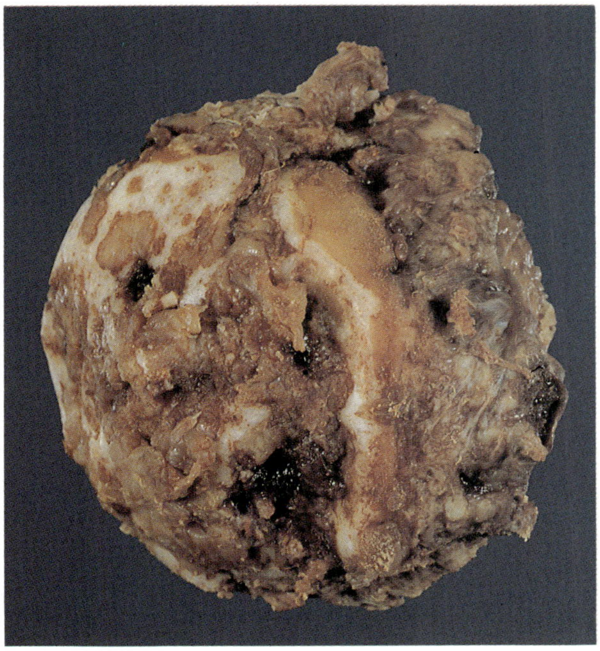

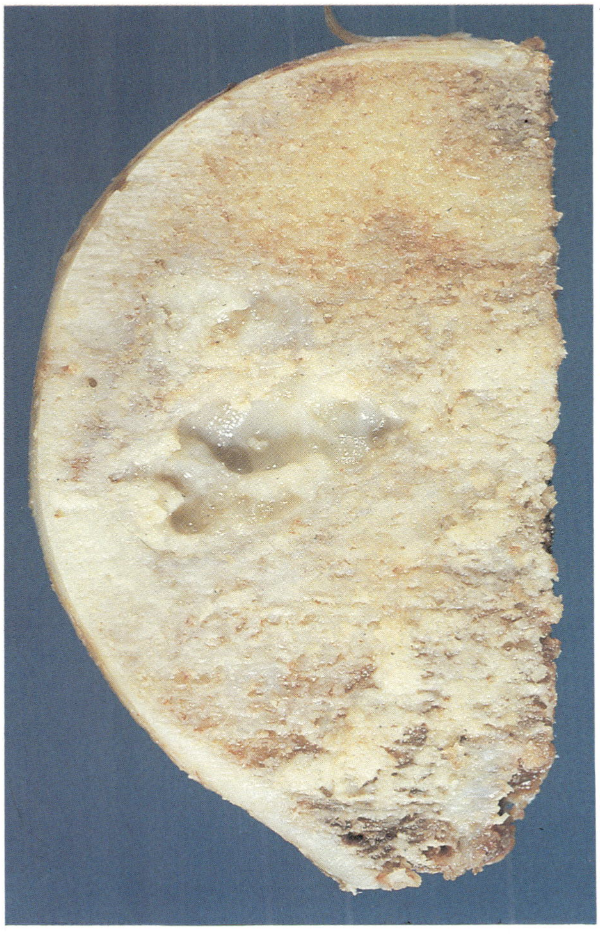

189

188 A femoral head from a patient with severe osteoarthritis of the hip. The articular cartilage has been largely lost, and the exposed underlying bone shows haemorrhagic discoloration.

189 A cross section of the bone in 188 showing eburnation of the articular surface and cyst formation in the subarticular bone.

Soft tissues

Skeletal muscle

Skeletal muscle biopsies are taken to investigate myopathies, myositis and denervation changes in muscle. The specimen should be sent fresh, as soon after removal as possible, held stretched either in a clamp or with sutures fixed to a wooden stick or board.

On receipt it is measured and described, (for example, 'A skeletal muscle biopsy measuring 4.1 × 1.2 × 1.3 cm received stretched along a tongue depressor. There is no apparent macroscopical abnormality'). Tissue is removed for freezing for enzyme histochemistry and fixation in glutaraldehyde for electron microscopy (crushed tissue adjacent to a clamp should be avoided). The remaining specimen is then pinned out onto a cork board and fixed fully. Transverse and longitudinal blocks are taken.

Soft tissue tumours

Soft tissue tumours of the extremities treated by amputation have been dealt with above. Tumours of the connective tissues of the thorax and abdomen include retroperitoneal liposarcoma and fibrosarcoma, mediastinal sarcomas, neurofibromas and neurofibrosarcomas, and vascular tumours. Soft tissue tumours are also relatively common in the skin and subcutis.

Dissection of specimen

The tumours may be excised with a rim of uninvolved adjacent tissues. The external surface of the specimen should be marked with India ink and photographs should be taken if possible. After measuring, the specimen should be sliced with a long-bladed knife at close intervals, and allowed to fix further if necessary (**190, 191**). The appearance of the tumour, its site of origin and its relation with the adjacent tissues should be recorded. Recognizable anatomical structures (such as oesophagus, thymus, inferior mesenteric vessels) should be examined to establish their relation to the tumour.

Example 190-191

The specimen consists of a multilobular mass of yellow adipose tissue measuring 12.2 × 13.5 × 8.4 cm. The external surface is smooth and glistening. The cut surface consists of rubbery uniform yellow tissue, the larger part of which is clearly defined and has a nodular pattern. In one area the edge of the tumour is indistinct and it appears to infiltrate adjacent fibrous tissue and skeletal muscle. In this infiltrative area there are several collections of clear myxoid material.

Blocks

- **A** centre of tumour × 2
- **B** myxoid area × 2
- **C** tumour and skeletal muscle × 2
- **D** excision margins × 5

190

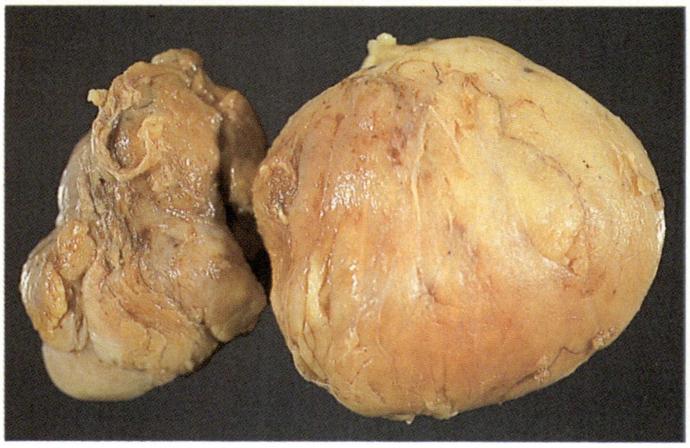

190 A tumour removed from the retroperitoneal area, found on microscopic examination to be a liposarcoma. Most of the tumour has a circumscribed outline with a smooth shiny surface, but part has an irregular outline and is covered by adherent skeletal muscle.

191

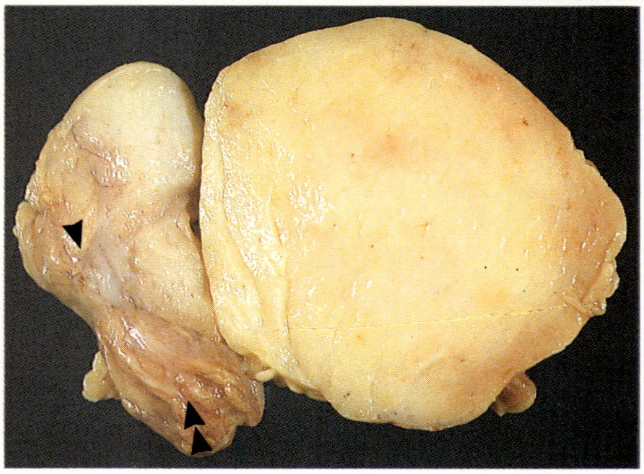

191 The cut surface of 190 showing soft yellow tissue with tiny haemorrhagic foci. Towards one edge there are foci of myxoid change (▶). The lesion infiltrates into adjacent skeletal muscle (▶▶).

CHAPTER 13
CARDIOVASCULAR SYSTEM

Small specimens

Vessels

Except in specialized centres, surgical removal of small or medium-sized arteries is seldom performed other than for the diagnosis of arteritis. Both temporal arteritis and polyarteritis nodosa affect arteries in a random and localized fashion, so it is important to examine as much of the tissue as possible. Small muscular arteries should be cut transversely at about 3 mm intervals and the blocks embedded 'on end'. Larger arteries removed during reconstructive surgery for atheroma can also be cut transversely and should be sampled along the length of the specimen. Blocks should be taken especially from areas where the media is replaced or expanded by gelatinous or soft yellow tissue, or where the intima is thickened or ulcerated. The macroscopical report is usually simple (for example, 'A cord of pale tissue measuring . . . . Bisected, both halves embedded, no reserve tissue', or 'A muscular artery measuring . . . cm long and . . . cm in diameter. 3 pieces'. If, however, there are localized dilatations, luminal thrombi or other focal lesions, these should also be mentioned.

Thrombosed superficial leg veins and haemorrhoids are occasionally sent for histological examination. Transverse blocks should be taken from cords of tissue, as for arteries. Haemorrhoidal veins are usually impossible to orientate and should be bisected or embedded whole. The measurements and descriptions are the same as for arteries.

Heart

Tiny biopsies of endocardium and immediately subjacent myocardium may be taken for investigation of transplant rejection. Pericardial biopsies may be received from cases of pericarditis or malignancy (usually mesothelioma). These are usually impossible to orientate, and are embedded whole. A very brief macroscopical report is generally sufficient (for example, 'An irregular fragment of pale tissue . . . . All embedded').

The macroscopical features of a diseased heart valve in most cases provide more information than its histology. If an entire valve or separate cusps are received, they should be measured, photographed and described (**192**). Representative transverse blocks should be taken for histology.

When fresh material is available, a small portion of each cusp should be sent for microbiological examination, especially when vegetations are present.

Heart valves: Macroscopical report	
Type of specimen	Mitral valve, semilunar valve cusp, irregular sheet of translucent tissue, etc.
Measurements	Diameter and circumference of valve ring if intact Number of cusps Size of aggregated specimen if fragmented
Description	Appearance of their surfaces, attachments and free edges, and presence of vegetations, holes, thickening, ulceration, calcification and fusion of commisures Condition of the cordae tendineae and attached papillary muscles

Large specimens

Entire hearts are very rarely received in pathology laboratories other than in specialist centres where heart transplantation is performed. The detailed protocols for examination of these specimens, developed within these specialized pathology departments, are outside the scope of this book.

Pericardium

Pericardiectomy specimens are taken for similar reasons to biopsies. They consist of irregular sheets of tissue, and are measured, described and blocked as for aneurysms, below.

Cardiac myxoma

Rarely, a round or ovoid gelatinous mass of cardiac myxoma may be excised from an atrium (**193**). The point of attachment to the endocardium can seldom be identified with confidence. After fixation and photography, parallel cuts are made through the specimen and several blocks of the myxoma are taken from areas with different macroscopical appearances (**194**).

Aneurysm sacs

Aneurysm sacs may be excised from the descending aorta or iliac vessels. The cut surface usually shows laminated thrombus within a degenerating elastic or muscular artery, but other tissues, such as muscle or fibrous tissue may form or be included in the aneurysm wall. After measurements have been taken and the tissue described briefly, several transverse sections should be made, and decalcified if necessary before processing.

Example 193-194

The specimen consists of a smooth-surfaced, soft multilobated mass of tissue measuring 9.5 × 6.1 × 4.5 cm and weighing 120 g. The cut surface shows soft, light-brown jelly-like tissue interspersed with areas of soft yellow material and foci of haemorrhage and necrosis.

Blocks × 4

Large cardiovascular specimens: Macroscopical report	
Type of specimen	Ovoid mass, sheet of pericardium, laminated thrombus and adjacent vessel wall
Measurements	Size of specimen (diameter or maximum dimension area and thickness)
Description	Colour Consistency (friable, gelatinous, hard, gritty, rubbery) Presence of adherent thrombus or clot

192 A mitral valve cusp with attached cordae, from a case of infective endocarditis. The cusp is thickened and opaque, and there are friable yellow vegetations on the atrial surface and free edge.

192

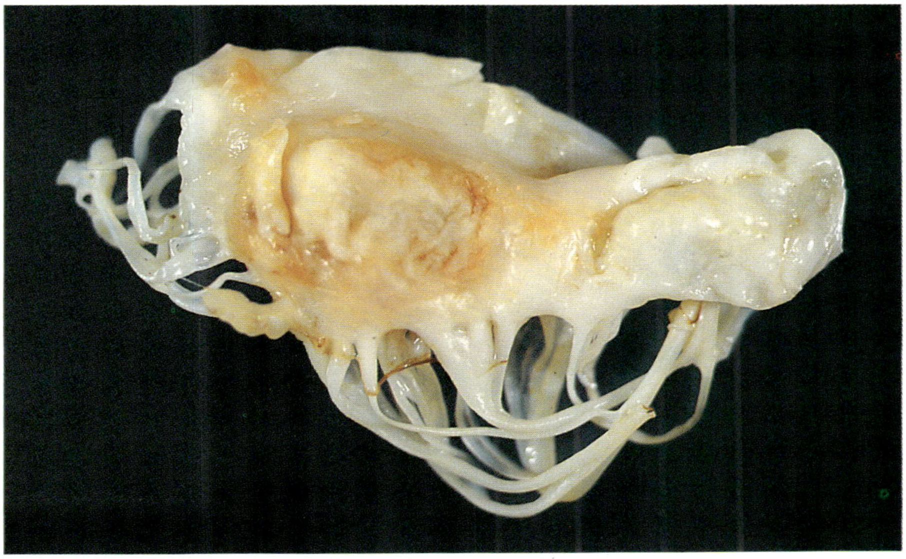

193 An atrial myxoma forming a smooth-surfaced, multilobated mass.

193

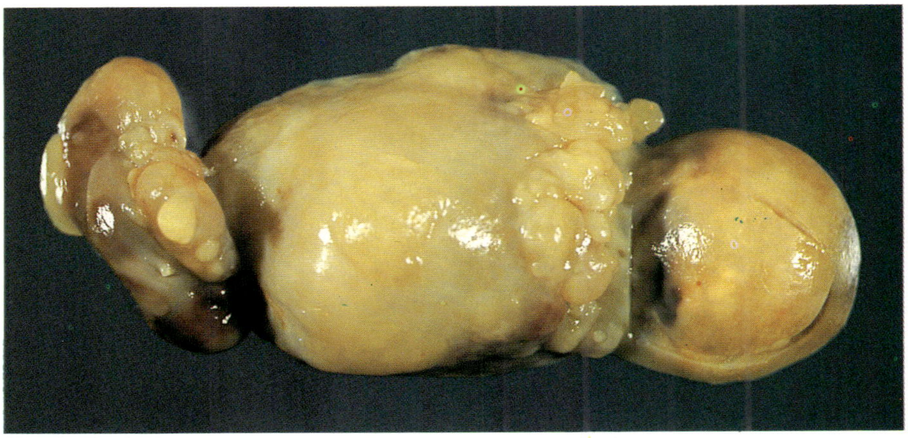

194 The cut surface of 193 showing light-brown jelly-like tissue interspersed with areas of soft yellow tissue and foci of haemorrhage.

194

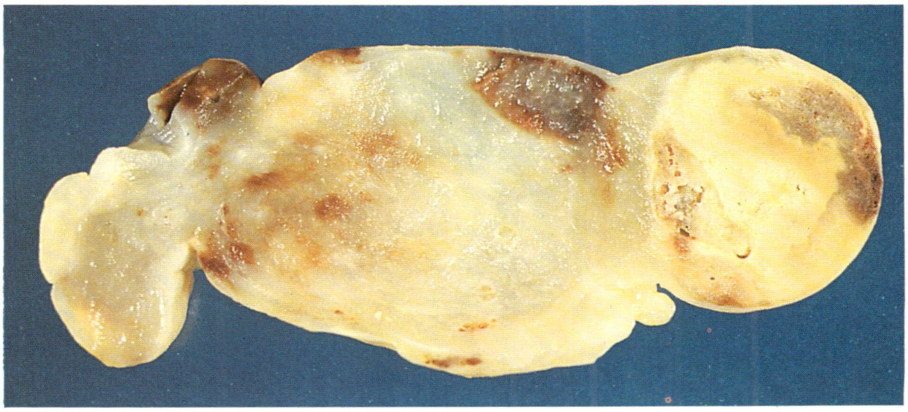

CHAPTER 14
CENTRAL NERVOUS SYSTEM AND EYE

Brain and meninges

Brain and meningeal biopsies are taken to investigate space-occupying lesions, and occasionally cerebral tissue is taken for diagnosis of inflammatory lesions such as viral encephalitis and some forms of dementia. Brain biopsies are usually small and may be fragmented. They are briefly described (for example, 'Irregular fragments of soft white tissue measuring . . .') and embedded in entirety. Larger pieces of cerebrum may also be received and will need slicing before blocks can be taken.

Meningiomas vary in size and may be received in fragmented form, but they often form large, rubbery, rounded masses of pink or grey tissue (**195**), in which case close parallel cuts should be made through the specimen. This allows the consistency to be assessed – if it is obviously gritty, the tissue should be decalcified before processing. The cut surface is usually homogeneous (**196**) and blocks can be taken from any area. If there are variegated areas, foci of haemorrhage or other tissues present, these should also be sampled.

195

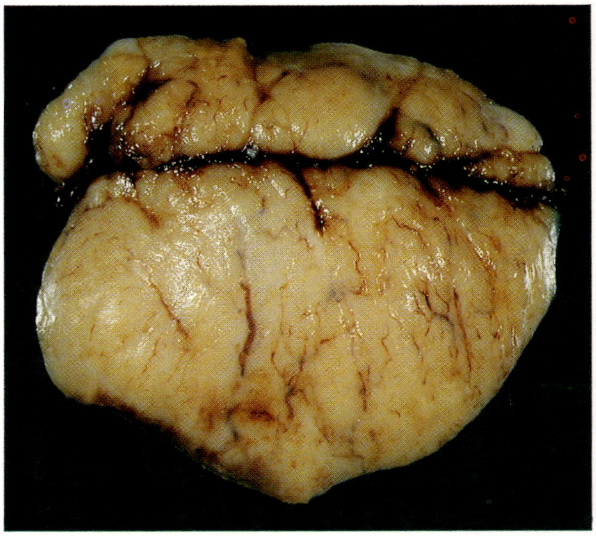

195 A meningioma removed by craniotomy. The tumour is a multinodular mass of rubbery tissue with a smooth surface.

196

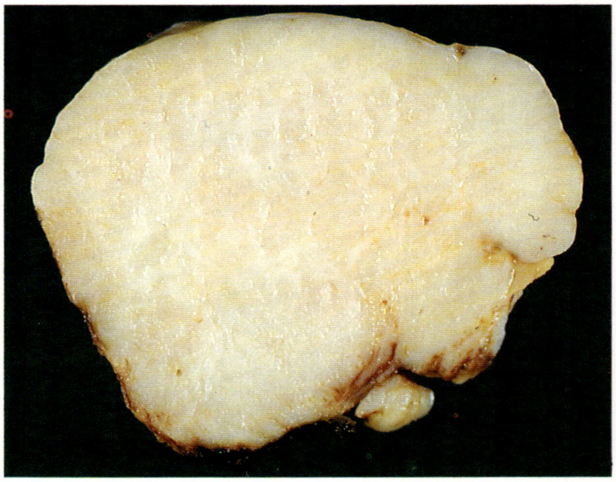

196 A slice from 195. The tumour tissue is white with a finely lobulated cut surface.

Peripheral nerves

Nerve trunks and ganglia may be received from vagotomy and sympathectomy operations. Histopathology is required simply to confirm the nature of the tissue. The entire specimen is cut into suitable lengths and embedded longitudinally. The macroscopical report consists of, for example, 'A cord of brown tissue 3 cm long and 0.2 cm in diameter. In the centre there is a fusiform enlargement 0.7 cm long and 0.5 cm in maximum diameter'.

Ocular biopsies: Macroscopical report	
Site of biopsy	This must always be recorded
Type of specimen	Tissue fragment, ellipse of skin, disc of tissue, mucosal biopsy, etc.
Measurements	Number of specimens Size in three planes, or greatest dimension if very small
Description	
Focal lesions	Size of nodules, pigmented patches, ulcers, etc., and their relation to excision margins
Rest of specimen	Colour and translucency; consistency (hard, firm, soft); presence of adherent adipose tissue or other structures

Eye

Biopsies

Biopsies may be taken from the conjunctiva, cornea, periorbital skin and soft tissues (including the eyelids and lacrimal gland) and from retro-orbital masses in order to investigate a variety of conditions including infection, other inflammatory conditions and neoplasia. Tissue may also rarely be removed from intraocular structures such as the iris, lens and trabecular meshwork for histological examination.

Most of these biopsies are small and delicate, and are fixed immediately after removal. As with any epithelial biopsy, it is essential that corneal and conjunctival biopsies are embedded 'on edge'. Most biopsies from the eye and periorbital tissues require no dissection and are embedded whole. Larger pieces of tissue should be bisected. Biopsies from the skin of the eyelids are treated as for skin elsewhere (p 97). The resection margins are usually identifiable on histological sections, but where this may be a problem the specimen should be marked with India ink.

Globes

Enucleation of the globe of the eye, leaving the eyelids and retrobulbar tissues *in situ*, may be carried out for intraocular tumours, trauma or severe intraocular inflammation, and if an eye is blind and painful. In cases of massive intraocular infection, evisceration may be performed instead; the contents of the globe are removed leaving the scleral envelope in place and the dural sheath around the optic nerve intact to reduce the risk of post-operative meningitis. Exenteration may be necessary for extensive conjunctival malignancy or for tumours involving the globe and extraocular tissues. This involves removal of the retrobulbar tissues and eyelids as well as the globe.

Dissection of globes

The dimensions of the eye, the diameter of the corneal disc and the length of the optic nerve attached to the back of the specimen should be measured. The globe is then fixed in formalin for at least 24 hours before dissection. Unless special procedures are intended, the specimen is left intact at this stage.

The eye can be orientated by the positions of the cut ends of the extraocular muscles relative to the position of the optic nerve (**197**). The external surface should be examined for evidence of trauma, scars and involvement by tumour. Before opening, it should be transilluminated with a strong point source of light to establish the size and position of any intraocular masses (**198, 199**). If a globe has been removed for malignant disease, tissue should be taken from the excision end of the optic nerve. The eye is then cut into three pieces called calottes, the most useful of which is an entire central cross section, about 8 mm thick, which includes the cornea and lens anteriorly and the optic nerve posteriorly (**200**). The plane of this central section is determined by the clinical history and the transillumination findings, and should include any focal lesion present. If there is none, or if an intraocular tumour occupies much of the globe, the eye should be cut in the horizontal plane.

Cutting the eye is best done with a fresh razor blade rather than a scalpel. After the globe has been orientated and transilluminated, it is placed cornea downwards, optic nerve upwards, on a pad of cotton wool. The first cut is then made vertically through the specimen about 2 mm to one side of the optic nerve down to the cornea just medial to the limbus. The globe can then be turned so that the cut surface is downwards on the cutting board, and a second cut is made parallel to the first to pass through the opposite limbus at the same level.

When the eye has been opened, the presence of tumours, retinal detachment and other lesions is noted and measurements are made.

Globes: Macroscopical report

Specimen	Right or left globe
Measurements	Anteroposterior, transverse and vertical dimensions, diameter of corneal disc, length of optic nerve
Description	
External	Clarity of cornea; size and shape of pupil, presence of synechiae; extraocular tumour involvement; adherent adipose tissue; suture markers on rectus muscles
Transillumination	Size, site and shape of shadows
Internal	Site, size, colour, consistency of focal lesions Vitreous body (tumour seeding, pus, foreign body) Retina (detachment, haemorrhage) Sclera (thinned, breached) Lens (focal opacities, cataracts) Ciliary body Anterior chamber (shallow, tumour deposits, presence of pus) Iris (coloboma, other defects)

Example 201-204

The specimen consists of a left globe measuring 2.3 cm vertically, 2.3 cm transversely and 2.5 cm anteroposteriorly. The corneal disc is transparent and 1.4 cm in diameter. The iris shows grade 4 arcus. The optic nerve is 1 cm long and 0.3 cm in diameter, and is surrounded by a moderate amount of adipose tissue. Within this fat there is a firm dark-brown nodule, 0.7 cm in maximum diameter and just inferomedial to the optic nerve, which is adherent to the external surface of the sclera.

Transillumination reveals a large defect to the passage of light occupying most of the posterior half of the globe.

On sectioning the eye, there is an irregular, large brown mass which has a broad-based attachment to most of the posterior wall. It measures 2.1 × 1.7 × 1.3 cm and bulges into the vitreous body, occupying approximately half of the volume of the posterior chamber. There is extensive retinal detachment overlying the tumour. The lens and anterior chamber appear macroscopically normal.

Blocks

A optic nerve resection margin × 1
B superior calotte × 1
C middle calotte × 1
D inferior calotte × 1
All embedded.

197 The orientation of a globe. The insertion of the superior oblique muscle (▶) is tendinous and lies superior and just lateral to the optic nerve (▶▶). The insertion of the inferior oblique muscle (▶▶▶) is muscular and lies inferior and lateral to the optic nerve. The superior and inferior rectus muscles (around which the opthalmic surgeon often places suture ties) lie on a perpendicular plane. This is therefore a right globe.

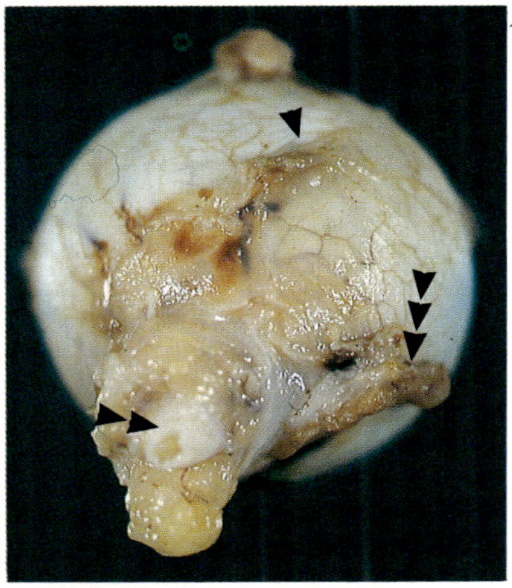

197

198 and **199** **The transillumination of a globe** to reveal intraocular masses. A strong point of light is held up against the globe, either to the sclera (**198**) or the cornea (**199**). If no masses are present between the light source and the aspect of the globe nearest the viewer, no shadows are seen. On rotation of the globe through 180° there is an interruption to the passage of light caused by a solid mass within the globe lying below the part nearest the viewer.

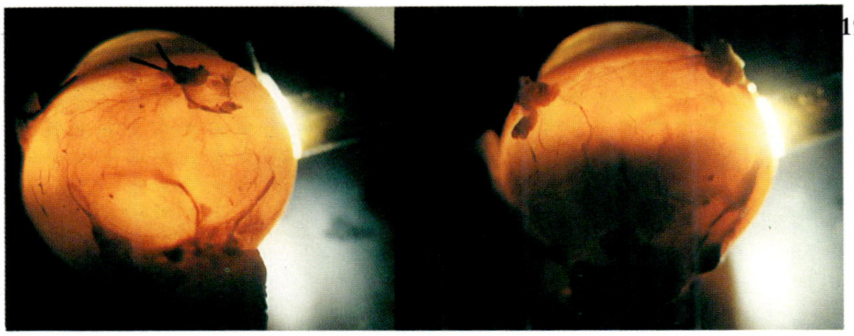

198

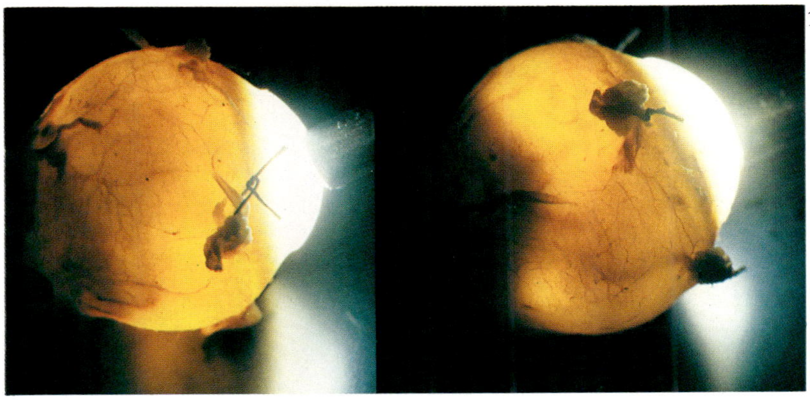

199

200 Central calotte from the left globe of a 2-year-old child. The grey tumour mass attached to the posterior surface of the retina overlying the optic disc is a retinoblastoma.

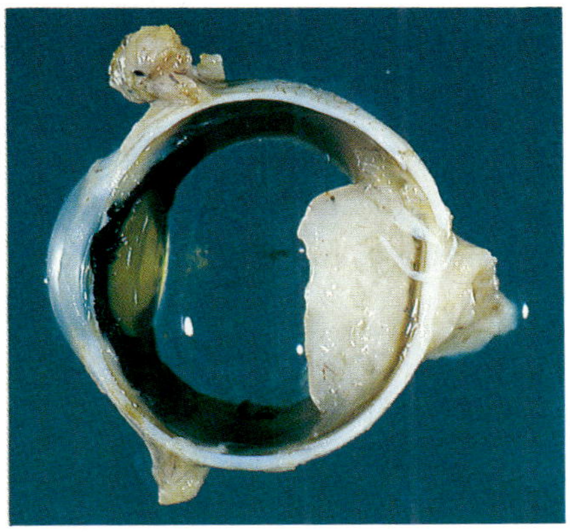

200

201

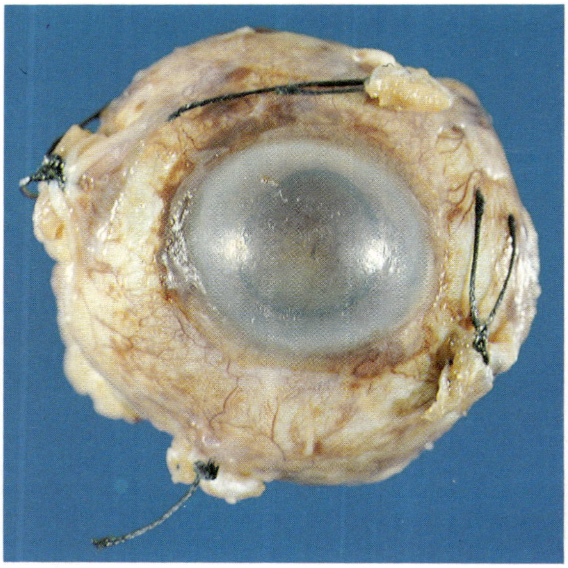

202

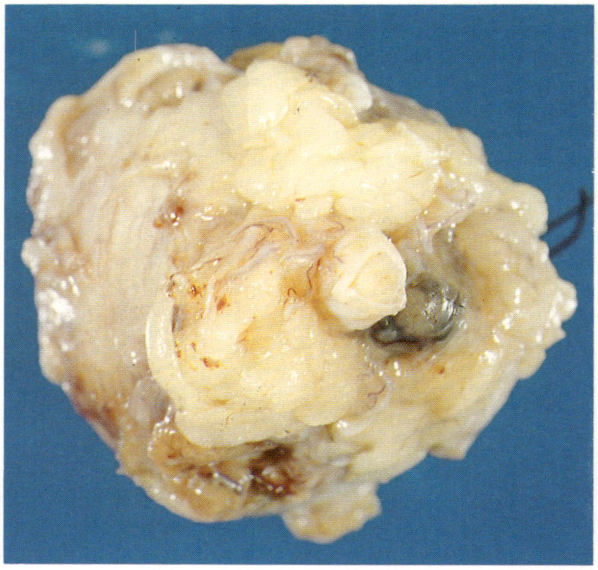

201 The anterior aspect of a left globe removed for choroidal melanoma.

202 The posterior aspect of 201 showing a pigmented extrasclerotic tumour nodule adjacent to the optic nerve.

203

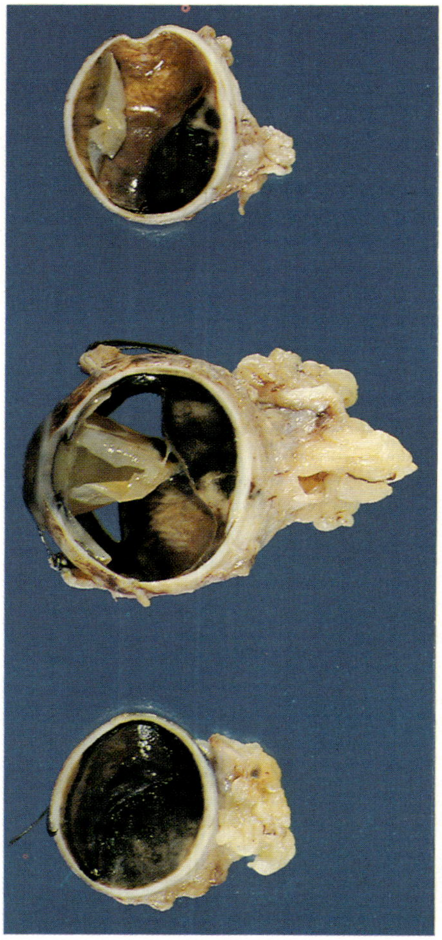

203 The globe in 201 and 202 divided into three horizontal calottes.

204 The other side of the central calotte from 203 showing a large choroidal melanoma attached to the posterior part of the globe, with overlying retinal detachment (▶). An extrascleral nodule is present in the orbital fat.

204

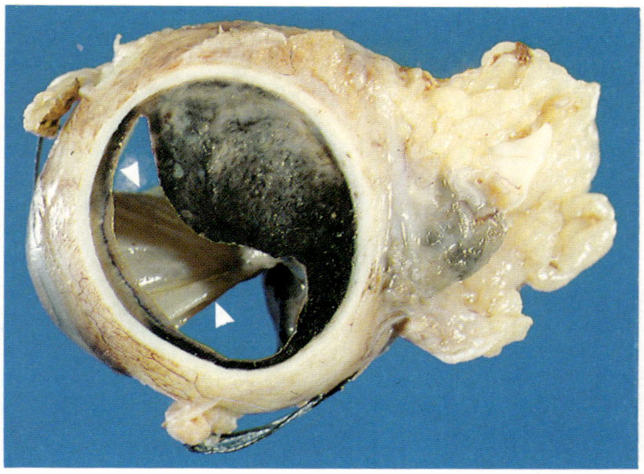

Index

All references are to page numbers

acetate strip 10, 12
adenoids 119-20
adrenal gland 107-9
— adenoma 107
— carcinoma 107
— ganglioneuroblastoma 107
— ganglioneuroma 107
— large specimens 107
— — dissection 107-8
— macroscopical report 108
— neuroblastoma 107
— phaeochromocytoma 107, 109
— small specimens 107
alimentary tract 10-30
— biopsies 10
— large bowel *see* large bowel
— large specimens 14
— polyps 11
— resection specimens 14
— small bowel *see* small bowel
— small lengths of wall 11
— small specimens 10
aneurysm sacs 134
appendicitis, acute purulent 23
appendix 21-3
— blocks 23
— dissection of specimen 21
— fibrosis of tip 22
— macroscopical report 22
— mucocele 22
— type of specimen 21
arteries 133
anus 28, 40, 41

bladder 87-91
— combined cystectomy-hysterectomy specimen 90
— fungating tumour 90
— large specimens 87
— — dissection 87-8
— macroscopical report on cystectomy specimen 88
— male patient 90, 91
— — blocks 91
— small specimens 87
blocks, general 8-9
— specific, *see under organ*
blood vessels 133
bone 124-31
— femoral heads 127
— fragments, specimens containing 9
— ischaemia, resection for 126
— — macroscopical report 127
— large specimens 124
— — dissection 124-6
— malignant disease, resection for 124-5
— — macroscopical report 125
— osteosarcoma 128
— small specimens 124
— specimens containing fragments 9
— trauma, resection for 126
— — macroscopical report 127
bone marrow 105
brain 136
breast 64-73
— biopsies 64-5
— — macroscopical report 64
— blocks from mastectomy specimen 71
— extended mastectomy specimen 70-1
— fibroadenoma 67
— intraduct papilloma 73
— large specimens 65-7
— — dissection 65-6
— — macroscopical report 66
— microcalcification 68
— multinodular papillomatous mass 73
— nipple dissection 73
— scirrhous carcinoma 72
— segmental mastectomy specimen 68-9
— simple mastectomy specimen 72
bronchial carcinoma 94
bronchiectasis 96
Buschke-Löwenstein tumour 80

calcification, specimens containing foci of 9
carcinoma cuniculatum 80
cartilage tumours 128, 129
cellulose acetate strip 10, 12
cervix 44-7
— biopsies 44
— — macroscopical report 44
— cone biopsy 44-7
— — dissection 44-5
— — macroscopical report 45
— — sequential slices 47
— curettings 44
choice of action 12
cholelithiasis 6
cholesterosis of gall bladder 33, 35
choroidal melanoma 140
cirrhosis 32, 33
coccyx 26
colectomy 25-29
colonic carcinoma blocks 29
condyloma of Buschke-Löwenstein 80
Crohn's disease 25
— differential diagnosis 6
cystectomy *see* bladder
cystic duct lymph node 34
decalcification 9
dissecting microscope 12, 82, 84

dissection principles 7-8
diverticular disease 26, 28-9
— blocks 27
doughnuts of bowel 11, 13
duodenum 36, 37
dysplasia, large bowel 30

ear 119
ectopic pregnancy 55, 56
EDTA 9
endometrium *see under* uterine corpus
epidermal cyst 99
epididymis 75
epididymitis, tuberculous 77
excision margins, markers for 9
eye 137-40
— choroidal melanoma 140
— biopsies 137
— — macroscopical report 137
— globes 137-8
— — macroscopical report 138
— — orientation 139
— — transillumination 139
— retinoblastoma 139

fallopian tube 55-6
— carcinoma 55
— ectopic pregnancy 55, 56
— macroscopical report 56
— sterilisation procedures 55
femoral head 127, 131
fetus 60, 61
— foot length/gestational age relationship 61
fibroids (leiomyomas) 48, 52, 55
— hysterectomy 50
— — macroscopical report 50
— intramural 55
— macroscopical report 48
— uterus with 55
— — blocks 55
fixation 5-6
fresh tissue 5

gall bladder 31, 33-5
— carcinoma 34
— cholesterosis 33, 35
— cystic duct lymph node 34
— dissection of specimen 33-4
— macroscopical report 34
gallstones 33, 35
ganglioneuroblastoma 107
ganglioneuroma 107
gastrectomy specimen 18-21
— blocks 21
— dissection of specimen 18-19
— — initial 18
— types 18
gestational sac 48, 51
giant condyloma of Buschke-Löwenstein 80
gingival cysts 119
glomus tumour 26
gout 127
Graves' disease, thyroid gland in 113

haemorrhoids 133
hairy cell leukaemia, spleen in 104
heart 133-5
— entire 134
— myxoma 134, 135
— valves 133, 135
hemicolectomy specimen 14
hepatocellular carcinoma 31, 32
Hirschsprung's disease, full thickness biopsies of bowel wall 11
Hodgkin's lymphoma, spleen in 103
hydatid disease of liver 31
hydatidiform mole 48, 52
hydronephrosis 86
hyperparathyroidism, primary 116
hysterectomy 48-55
— extended 49
— for: carcinoma 49-50, 54
— — fibroids 50, 55
— — non-neoplastic disease 50-1
— macroscopical report 50
— Wertheim's 49

ischaemic colitis 25
ink marker for resection margins 9

jejunal biopsies 10
joint lesions 127

kidney 82-6
— blocks from nephrectomy specimen 85
— carcinoma 82, 83
— — metastasis in lung 95
— — nephrectomy for 82-3, 86
— hydronephrotic 86
— large specimens 82-4
— — dissection 82-3
— macroscopical report 83
— needle biopsy 82, 84
— non-neoplastic disease, nephrectomy for 83
— renal pelvic mass 85
— small specimens 82

labial cysts 119
large bowel 12, 25-30
— biopsies 12
— blocks 14, 27
— pedunculated polyp 13
— plaque-like tumour 29
— rectal biopsy 12
— rings excised 13
— sessile polyp 13
larynx 120-2
— angiosarcoma 122
— laryngectomy specimens 120-3

— macroscopical report 120
leiomyomas *see* fibroids
lingual cyst 119
liposarcoma 132
liver 31-3
— blocks 33
— cirrhosis 33
— dissection of specimen 31-3
— large specimen 31
— macroscopical report 31
— small specimen 31
lower limbs, blood supply 130
lungs 92-6
— bronchiectasis 96
— large specimen 92
— macroscopical report 93
— renal carcinoma metastasis 95
— small specimen 92
lymph nodes 101-2
— abdominal 14-15, 27
— macroscopical report 101
lymphoma 101-4
— Hodgkin's disease 103
— lymphoplasmacytoid 102

macroscopical description 6-7
macroscopical reports *see specific organs*
Meckel's diverticulum 21-3, 24
— blocks 23
— dissection of specimen 21
— macroscopical report 22
— type of specimen 21
meninges 136
meningioma 136
Merkel cell tumour (neuroendocrine tumour of skin) 100
methyl green pyronin stain 9
morphological terms 7
muscle biopsy, skeletal 132

nephrectomy, for:
— carcinoma 82
— non-neoplastic disease 83
nerve trunks/ganglia 136
neuroblastoma 107
neuroendocrine tumour of skin (Merkel cell tumour) 100
nose
— inverted squamous cell papilloma (Ringert's tumour; Schneiderian papilloma; transitional cell papilloma) 119
— macroscopical report 119
— polyps 119, 121

oesophagectomy 15-17
— blocks 17
— dissection 15-16
— — initial 15
— macroscopical report 16
— types of specimen 15
oesophagogastrectomy 18
oesophagus 15-17
— carcinoma 17
oral cavity 119
— cysts 119
osteosarcoma 128
ovary 57-9
— carcinoma 59
— cyst 58, 59
— large specimens 57-8
— — dissection 57-8
— macroscopical report 57
— small specimens 57
— solid tumour 59

pancreas, endocrine 117-18
— blocks from partial pancreatectomy 118
— islet cell neoplasms 117, 118
— macroscopical report 117
pancreas, exocrine 36-9
— large specimens 36-7
— — dissection 36-7
— macroscopical report 37
— small specimens 36
— Whipple's operation specimen 36-9
— — blocks 38
pancreatectomy 36, 117
para-articular tissues 127
parathyroid glands 115-16
— macroscopical report 116
penis 80-1
— macroscopic report 80
— squamous cell carcinoma 80
peptic ulcer, perforated 19
periampullary carcinoma 37
pericardial biopsy 133, 134
perineum 40-42
peripheral nerves 136
Perls' stain 9
phaeochromocytoma 107, 109
pharyngeal pouch 120, 121
photography 5
pigments for marking resection margins 9
pituitary gland 107
placenta 60-3
— intervillous fibrin deposition 63
— twin pregnancy 62
pleura 92-6
— large specimen 93
— macroscopical report 93
— small specimens 92
— tumour infiltration 96
polyarteritis nodosa 133
polyps
— gastrointestinal 11, 12, 26
— — pedunculated 13
— — sessile 13

— nasal 119, 121
prepatellar bursa 131
principles of dissection 7
prostate 77-9
— adenocarcinoma 79
— benign nodular hyperplasia 79
— large specimens 78
— macroscopical report 78
— multinodular masses 79
— small specimens 77-8
— weight 6
protocolectomy specimen 25

rectum
— abdominoperineal resection 27
— biopsy 12
— carcinoma 26, 27, 28
— combined anteroposterior resection 24
— villous adenomas 26
renal parenchymal cell carcinoma 82, 83
resection margins, markers for 9
retinoblastoma 139
Ringert's tumour 119
rubber stamp 12

salivary glands 123
salpingitis 55
Schneiderian papilloma 119
scrotum 80-1
sialolithiasis 6
skeletal muscle biopsy 132
skin 97-100
— bulla 98
— epidermal cyst 99
— intradermal nodule 99
— macroscopical report 97
— Merkel cell tumour (neuroendocrine tumour of skin) 100
— pigmented lesion 99
— tumour, blocks from 99
— vesicle 98
skull, metastatic thyroid follicular carcinoma tumour 129, 130
small bowel 25-7
— dissecting microscope view 12
— dissection 25-7
— macroscopical report 26
— types of specimen 25
soft tissue tumours 132
specimen identification 5
spleen 102-3
— dissection 102
— in: hairy cell leukaemia 104
— Hodgkin's lymphoma 103
— macroscopical report 102
sterilisation procedures 55
stomach 18-21
— carcinoma 20
— specimens 18, 20
— — perforated 19
see also gastrectomy

temporal arteritis 133
testis 74-5, 76-7
— large specimens 74
— — dissection 74-5
— macroscopical report 75
— small specimens 74
thymus 105-6
— macroscopical report 105
thyroid gland 110-15
— blocks 112
— carcinoma 114-15
— in Graves' disease 113
— large specimens 110
— — dissection 110
— macroscopical report 111
— multinodular goitre 113-14
— nodule 112
— small specimens 110
tonsils 119-20

ulcerative colitis 25, 30
— differential diagnosis 6
unfixed tissue 5
ureter 87
uterine corpus 48-55
— chorionic villi 48
— endometrium 48
— — macroscopical report 48
— fibroids *see* fibroids
— large specimens 48-9
— — dissection 49
— small specimens 48
— *see also* hysterectomy

vas deferens 75
veins
— haemorrhoidal 133
— thrombosed, of leg 133
vulva 40-3
— blocks from vulvectomy specimen 43
— carcinoma 41
— large specimens 40-3
— — dissection 40-1
— macroscopical report 40
— nodular tumour 41
— small specimens 40

weights of organs and tissues 6
Wertheim's hysterectomy specimen 49, 50
Whipple's operation specimen 36-8